Mediterranean Delights

A Collection of Easy & Tasty Recipes for Your Mediterranean Meals

Emma Kirk

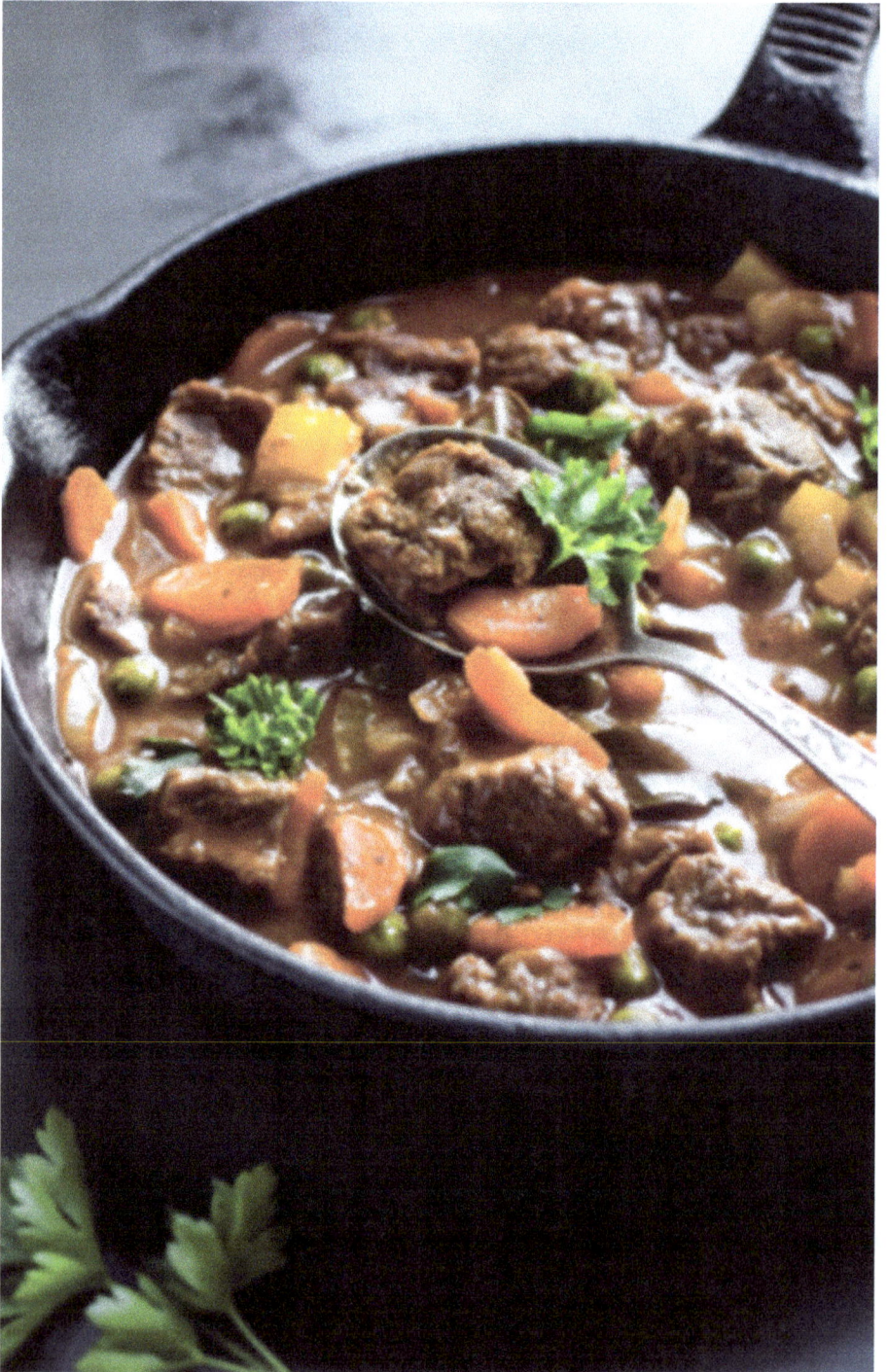

By reading this document, the reader agrees that under no circumstances is the author responsible for any losses, direct or indirect, which are incurred as a result of the use of information contained within this document, including, but not limited to, — errors, omissions, or inaccuracies.

Table of Contents

5

Mediterranean grain bowl recipe with lentils and chickpeas

Ingredients

- 2 ½ tablespoons of fresh lemon juice
- Salt
- 1 zucchini squash, sliced into rounds
- 3 cups cooked faro
- 2 cups of cooked brown lentils
- 2 cups of cooked chickpeas
- ½ teaspoons of ground Sumac
- 2 ½ teaspoons of quality Dijon mustard
- 1 teaspoon of Za'atar spice
- Extra virgin olive oil
- 2 cups of cherry tomatoes, halved
- 2 shallots, sliced
- 1 cup of fresh chopped parsley
- Handful pitted Kalamata olives
- Sprinkle of crumbled feta cheese
- 2 avocados, skin removed, pitted and sliced
- 1 garlic clove, minced
- Salt and pepper

Directions

- In a skillet, heat 2 tablespoons of olive oil over medium heat until shimmering but without smoke.
- Add the sliced zucchini and sauté on both sides until tender.
- Remove zucchini and place on a paper towel to drain any excess oil.
- Season with salt.

- Add the extra virgin olive oil, lemon juice, garlic, salt and pepper, za'atar spice, and sumac to a mason jar.
- Close tightly, and give it a good shake. Set aside for later.
- Divide the cooked faro, lentils, and chickpeas equally among four dinner bowls.
- Add cooked zucchini, tomatoes, shallots, avocado slices, parsley, and Kalamata olives.
- Season with salt, pepper and za'atar then drizzle a bit of the dressing on top.
- Serve and enjoy at room temperature.

Roasted cauliflower and chickpea stew

This is a perfect match for serving over couscous or rice. The cauliflower is deliciously roasted and loaded with carrots, cumin, tomatoes, cinnamon and paprika for a Mediterranean dish.

Ingredients

- ½ cup of parsley leaves, stems removed, roughly chopped
- 1 ½ teaspoons of ground turmeric
- 1 28-oz. can of diced tomatoes with its juice
- 1 ½ teaspoons of ground cumin
- 1 ½ teaspoons of ground cinnamon
- 1 teaspoon of Sweet paprika
- Toasted pine nuts
- 2 14-oz. cans of chickpeas, drained and rinsed
- 1 teaspoon of cayenne pepper
- ½ teaspoon of ground green cardamom
- 1 whole head cauliflower, divided into small florets
- 5 medium-sized bulk carrots, peeled, cut pieces
- Salt and pepper
- Extra virgin olive oil
- Toasted slivered almonds
- 1 large sweet onion, chopped
- 1 teaspoon of ground coriander
- 6 garlic cloves, chopped

Directions

- Preheat the oven to 475°F.
- In a small bowl, mix together the spices.

- Place the cauliflower florets and carrot pieces on a large lightly oiled baking sheet.
- Season with salt and pepper.
- Add some spice mixture.
- Drizzle with olive oil, then toss to coat.
- Bake for 20 minutes in the preheated oven or until the carrots and cauliflower soften.
- Remove from the heat and keep for later. Turn the oven off.
- In a large cast iron pot , heat 2 tablespoons of olive oil.
- Add the onions and sauté for 3 minutes, add the garlic and the remaining spices.
- Let cook for 3 minutes on medium-high heat, stirring constantly.
- Add chickpeas with the canned tomatoes.
- Season with salt and pepper.
- Stir in the roasted cauliflower and carrots boil.
- Lower the heat, cover part-way let cook for 20 minutes.
- Transfer to serving bowls and garnish with fresh parsley.
- Serve and enjoy place over couscous.

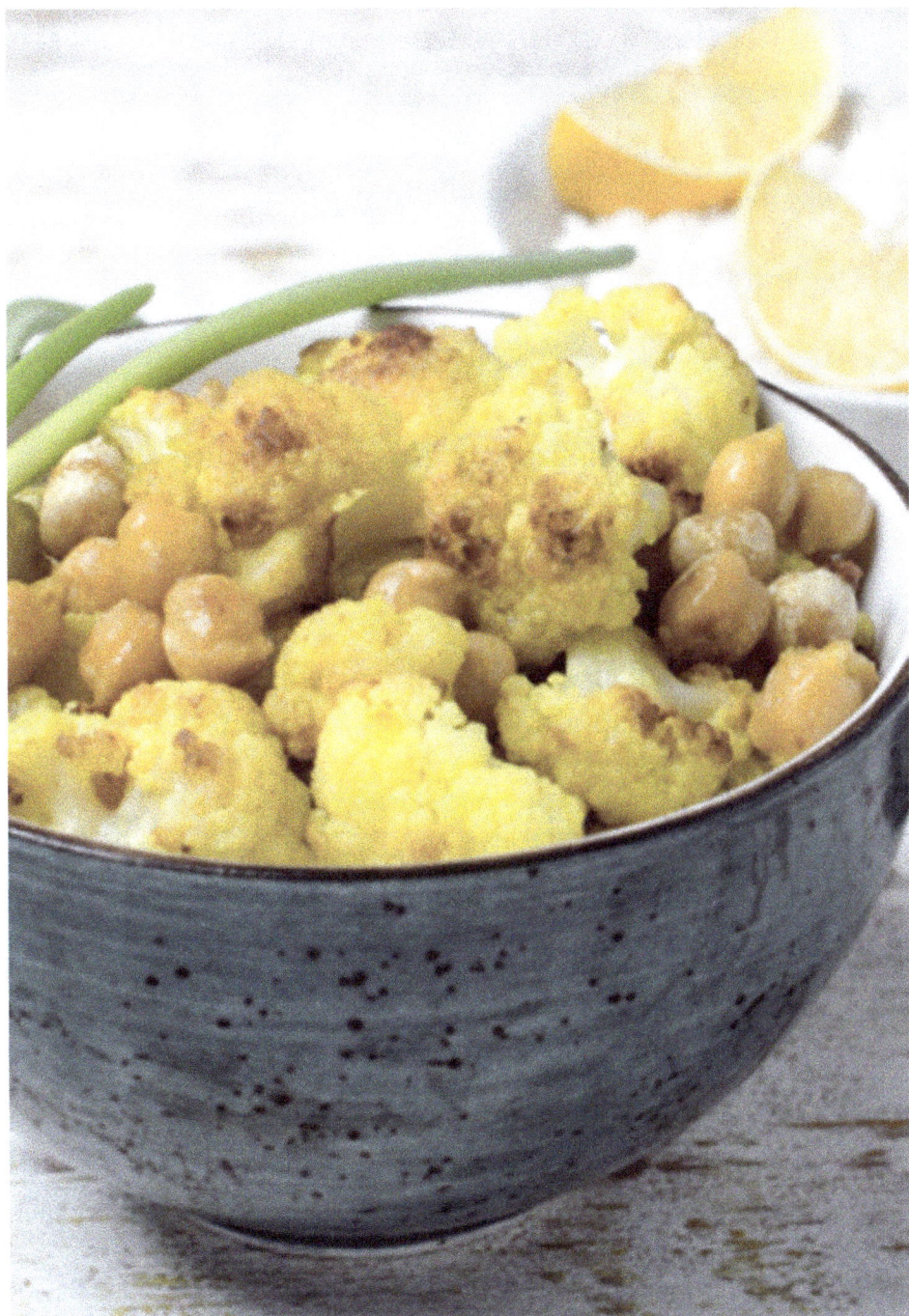

Jeweled couscous recipe with pomegranate and lentils

This recipe combines mushrooms, lentil, nuts and raisins for a gorgeous dish the Mediterranean Sea way for a vegan.

Ingredients

- Salt
- ½ teaspoon of turmeric spice
- Olive oil
- 8 oz. mushrooms, cleaned and sliced
- 3 garlic cloves, chopped
- 1 teaspoon of sweet paprika
- 1 ⅔ cup of vegetable broth
- Water
- ½ teaspoon of ground green cardamom
- ½ teaspoon of ground coriander
- 1 cup of lentils
- 1 cup of gold raisins
- ½ cup of shelled chopped pistachios
- ½ teaspoon of ground cumin
- 2 cups of instant couscous
- 1 bunch of fresh mint stems removed, chopped
- ½ teaspoon of freshly ground black pepper
- 2 tablespoons of pomegranate molasses
- Juice of ½ lemon
- 1 bunch of fresh parsley, stems removed, chopped
- 1 small red onion, chopped
- 1 ½ teaspoon of ground cinnamon
- 6 scallions, tops trimmed, chopped
- Seeds of 1 large pomegranate

- 10 Medjool dates , pitted, chopped

Directions

- Wash the lentils under running water. Drain.
- Place the lentils in a saucepan and add 3 cups of water let boil, then reduce to simmer for 30 minutes.
- Add a pinch of salt and remove from heat.
- In a saucepan, bring the vegetable broth to a boil.
- Stir in couscous together with the turmeric, pinch of salt, olive oil.
- Cover and let sit 5 minutes to finish cooking.
- In a large cast iron skillet, heat 2 tablespoons of olive oil.
- Add the mushrooms let cook for 4 minutes on high, tossing occasionally.
- Reduce heat to medium-high, and stir the onions and garlic and cook briefly.
- In the same skillet, add in the cooked lentils and couscous.
- Add salt together with the cinnamon, cardamom, paprika, coriander, and black pepper.
- Mix the pomegranate molasses and lemon juice with 1 tablespoon of olive oil.
- Add the liquid to the skillet with the couscous and lentil mixture. Toss to combine.
- Let cook on medium, stirring regularly to warm through.
- Remove from the heat, add the remaining ingredients.
- Move the couscous to a serving platter.

- Serve and enjoy.

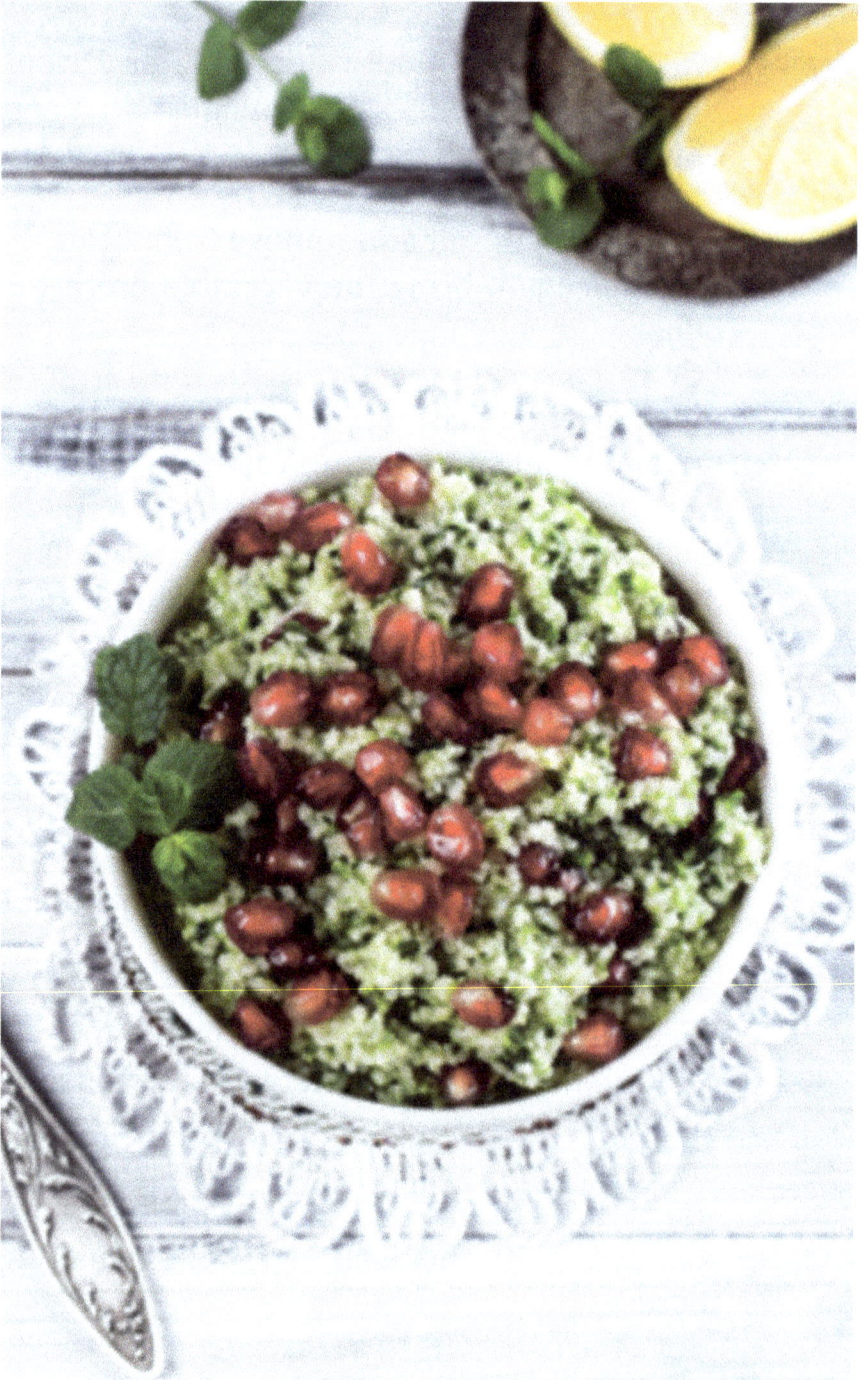

Easy Mediterranean style shrimp stew

This easy Mediterranean shrimp stew is prepared with chunky yet rustic tomato sauce with wonderful flavor from the garlic, onions, and bell peppers.

Ingredients
- ⅓ cup of toasted pine nuts, optional
- 1 large red onion, chopped
- 1 ½ teaspoon of ground coriander
- 1 bell pepper, cored, chopped
- 5 garlic cloves, chopped
- ¼ cup of toasted sesame seeds
- 1 teaspoon of sumac
- Extra virgin olive oil
- Lemon or lime wedges
- 1 teaspoon of red pepper flakes
- ½ teaspoon of ground green cardamom
- 2 15-oz. cans of diced tomatoes
- ½ cup water
- Kosher salt and black pepper
- 1 teaspoon of cumin
- 2 ½ lb. large shrimp
- 1 cup of parsley leaves

Directions
- Preheat the oven to 375°F.
- In a large skillet or frying pan, heat 2 tablespoons of extra virgin olive oil until shimmering but with smoke.
- Add chopped onions, bell peppers, and garlic.
- Let cook for 4 minutes, tossing regularly.
- Stir in spices and continue to cook for 1 more minute.

- Add diced tomatoes and water.
- Season with kosher salt and pepper.
- Boil, then lower heat to let simmer 15 minutes.
- Transfer sauce to an oven-save dish.
- Stir shrimp into the sauce.
- Add parsley together with the pine nuts, and toasted sesame seeds.
- Tighten the lid with a foil.
- Transfer to heated oven let bake for 9 minutes.
- Uncover and broil briefly till shrimp is ready.
- Serve and enjoy.

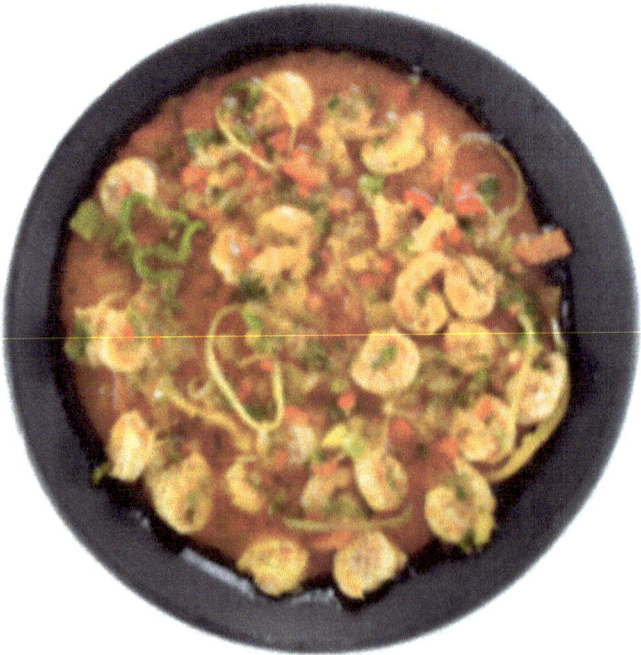

Extra creamy avocado hummus recipe

Avocado is the king for skin nourishing among Mediterranean Sea diet recipes. Chickpeas combined with creamy avocado will definitely surprise your taste buds every possible way flavored with garlic, cumin and cayenne.

Ingredients

- ½ lime, juice of lemon
- 2 garlic cloves
- 15-oz. can of chickpeas, drained
- Liquid from canned chickpeas
- ½ teaspoon of cayenne pepper
- 2 tablespoons of Greek Yogurt
- 3 tablespoons of tahini
- Salt
- 2 medium ripe avocados, roughly chopped
- 1 teaspoon of ground cumin

Directions

- In a large food processor, add the garlic together with the chickpeas, avocados, Greek yogurt, tahini, salt, cumin, cayenne and lime juice.
- Blend until the hummus mixture is smooth.
- Taste and adjust everything accordingly.
- Run the processor again until you achieve the desired creamy consistency. Again adjust seasoning as required.
- Transfer the avocado hummus to a serving dish and cover tightly with plastic wrap.
- Chill in a refrigerator before serving.

- Uncover and smooth the surface of the hummus and drizzle a bit of extra virgin olive oil.
- Garnish with fresh parsley.
- Serve and enjoy.

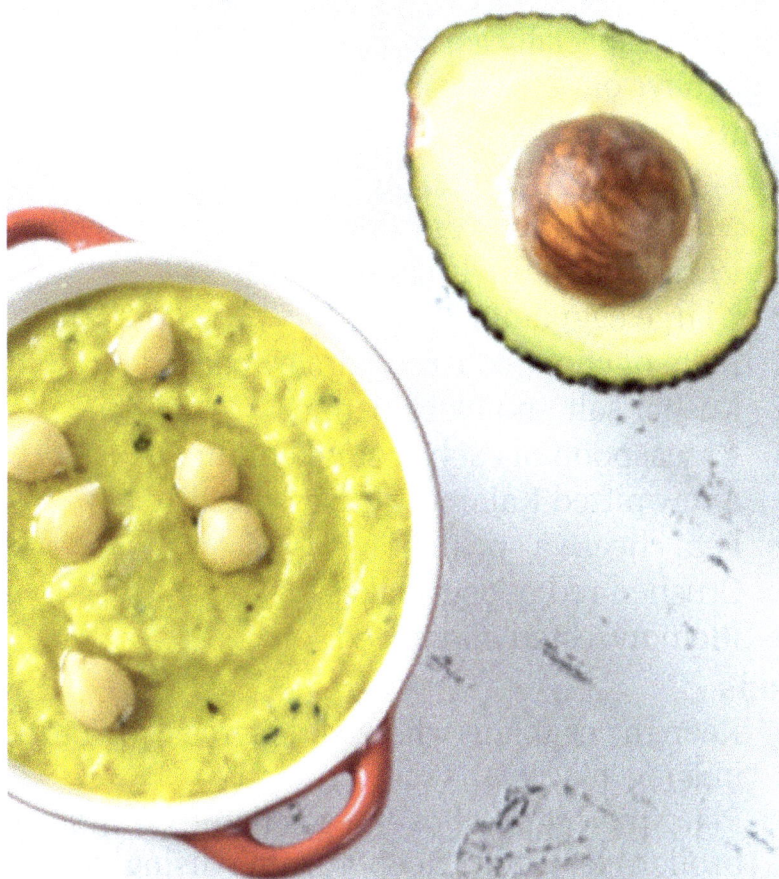

Melitzanosalata recipe

This recipe copes the Greek style of smoky dip of eggplant with aromatics especially garlic, parsley, lemon juice, and extra virgin olive oil.

Ingredients

- ¼ cup of [extra virgin olive oil](extra%20virgin%20olive%20oil)
- 2 large garlic cloves minced
- ¼ red onion finely chopped
- 2 large eggplants
- 1 cup of chopped fresh parsley packed
- Kosher salt and black pepper
- ½ teaspoon of each ground cumin
- A few pitted Kalamata olives sliced
- Feta cheese a sprinkle
- Crushed red pepper flakes
- 1 lemon zested and juiced

Directions

- Keep the eggplant whole and pierce with a fork in a few places.
- Place the eggplant over a gas flame or under a broiler, let cook, keep turning using tongs, until the skin is fully charred
- Cool and drain eggplant.
- Place the eggplant in a bowl and until cool enough to handle.
- Peel the charred skins off and discard.
- Cut into chunks and place in a colander to get rid of any remaining excess juices for 10 minutes.
- Shift eggplant to a mixing bowl.

- Add the <u>garlic together with the onion, parsley, lemon juice, olive oil</u> .
- Add salt and pepper and spices, mix to combine.
- Break up the eggplant into smaller chunks.
- Cover the eggplant dip well, let chill in the refrigerator shortly.
- Transfer the eggplant dip to a serving plate and spread.
- Drizzle with extra virgin olive oil.
- Organize and garnish with red onions, lemon zest, parsley, olives, a sprinkle of feta.
- Serve and enjoy with crusty bread.

Veggie teriyaki stir-fry with noodles

Quick and easy stir fry vegetables with noodles for a healthy dinner is perfect for a Mediterranean Sea diet in 40 minutes max.

Ingredients

- ½ cup [teriyaki sauce](#)
- ¼ cup thinly sliced green onion
- 2 tablespoons extra-virgin olive oil
- ½ teaspoon fine sea salt
- 6 cups thinly sliced mixed vegetables*
- 1 to 2 teaspoons toasted sesame oil
- 1 medium red or white onion
- 4 ounces soba noodles, brown rice noodles
- 1 teaspoon sesame seeds

Directions

- Bring a pot of water to boil.
- Place the noodles let cook the noodles as per the package Directions.
- Drain and set aside for later.
- Warm a large skillet over medium heat.
- Add the oil, onion, and salt let for 4 – 6 minutes until onions are tender.
- Add the remaining vegetables and cook until they are tender and caramelizing on the edges in 10 – 15 minutes.
- Add the noodles and ½ cup of teriyaki sauce to the pan.
- Stir to combine, let cook till the ingredients are all warmed through in 1 minute.
- Remove the skillet from the heat source.

- Add toasted sesame oil together with the sesame seeds.
- Serve the noodles in bowls with sliced green onion.
- Sprinkle with sesame seeds on top.
- Serve and enjoy.

Roasted butternut squash, pomegranate and wild rice stuffing

The recipe can take up to 1 hour and 20 minutes but the sweetness and the health benefit achieved from eating it makes it worth waiting for. It is prepared with kale, wild rice and pomegranate serving from 6 – 12 servings.

Ingredients

- Arils from 1 medium pomegranate,
- 1 tablespoon of maple syrup
- 1 tablespoon of Dijon mustard
- 4 ounces of kale, ribs removed and chopped
- ¾ cup of chopped green onion
- 1 tablespoon of grated fresh ginger
- ½ cup of raw pepitas
- 1 teaspoon of extra-virgin olive oil
- 2 teaspoon of fine sea salt
- 2 tablespoons of apple cider vinegar
- 2 cups of wild rice
- ¼ teaspoon ground cinnamon
- 1 small-to-medium butternut squash
- 2 teaspoon of fine sea salt
- 4 ounces of goat cheese
- ¼ cup of extra-virgin olive oil

Directions

- Preheat your oven to 425°F.
- Line a large baking sheet with parchment paper.
- Bring a large pot of water to boil.
- Add the rice let cook under reducing heat to simmer for 40 – 55 minutes.

- Remove from heat, drain, return the rice to the pot
- Place the cubed butternut squash onto the baking sheet.
- Drizzle it with the olive oil and a sprinkle of salt.
- Toss until the cubes are lightly and evenly coated in oil.
- Arrange them in single layer let roast for 35 – 50 minutes tossing occasionally.
- Chop the kale and green onion, remove the arils from the pomegranate, whisk together dressing ingredients in a small bowl.
- combine the pepitas with 1 teaspoon olive oil, ¼ teaspoon of salt and cinnamon in a small skillet stir. Cook for 3 – 5 minutes.
- Stir in half of the green onions, kale, and ginger dressing.
- Spread the mixture over a large serving platter.
- Arrange the butternut squash over the wild rice mixture.
- Crumble the goat cheese on top with a fork.
- Top with the toasted pepitas, pomegranate arils, and green onions.
- Serve while warm and enjoy.

Crispy bean tostadas with smashed avocado and jicama-cilantro slaw

The beans are refried the Mexican way with avocado and cabbage slaw crisp. Prepared with fillings entirely meatless perfect for a Mediterranean Sea diet.

Ingredients

- ½ medium red onion, thinly sliced
- Salt
- Juice of 2 lime
- 6 corn of tortillas
- 2 cups shredded green cabbage
- ½ cup of crumbled queso fresco
- ½ teaspoon ground cumin
- Freshly ground black pepper
- ½ cup fresh cilantro leaves
- Extra-virgin olive oil
- 2 cans of vegetarian refried beans
- 1 tablespoon white vinegar
- ½ teaspoon chili powder
- 3 large ripe avocados, pitted and peeled
- ½ cup ¼-inch-thick slices peeled jicama
- ½ cup of halved grape tomatoes

Directions

- In a medium bowl, combine the sliced onions together with the lime juice, vinegar and salt stir to coated the onions set aside.
- In a large bowl, combine the cilantro, cabbage, lime juice, jicama, cumin and chili powder.
- Season with salt and pepper accordingly.
- Preheat your oven to 425°F.

- Brush both sides of the tortilla with olive oil let season with salt.
- Organize in a single layer on a large baking sheet.
- Bake for 4 minutes, flip and bake for 4 – 8 minutes, till crispy.
- Gently heat the refried beans in the microwave.
- In a large sized bowl, mash the avocados with a fork.
- Stir in the lime juice and season with salt accordingly.
- Spread refried beans evenly over every tortilla.
- Add a layer of smashed avocado and top with the pickled onions, slaw, tomatoes and queso fresco.
- Serve soon enough and enjoy.

Mango burrito bowls with crispy tofu and peanut sauce

The recipe is prepared with tofu, brown rice, peanut sauce and fresh mango from the tree. It takes max I hour and 15 minutes to get ready.

Ingredients

- ½ cup of sliced green onions
- 1 block of organic extra-firm tofu
- 1 medium red bell pepper, chopped
- 1 tablespoon extra-virgin olive oil
- ¼ cup chopped fresh cilantro
- 3 tablespoon reduced-sodium tamari
- 2 cups shredded cabbage
- ¼ teaspoon fine sea salt
- 1 tablespoon cornstarch
- 1 medium jalapeño, seeds and ribs removed, minced
- 1 ¼ cups brown basmati rice
- ⅓ cup creamy peanut butter
- 5 tablespoons lime juice
- 1 tablespoon honey or maple syrup, to taste
- 2 teaspoons toasted sesame oil
- Handful of chopped roasted peanuts
- 2 garlic cloves, minced
- ¼ teaspoon red pepper flakes
- 2 large ripe mangos

Directions

- Preheat your oven to 400°F.
- Align a large baking sheet with parchment paper.
- Drain the tofu.

- Slice the tofu into thirds lengthwise in 3 even slabs.
- Stack the slabs on top of each other and slice through them lengthwise to 3 even columns, slice across to 5 even rows.
- Arrange the tofu in an even layer on a board with towels.
- Fold the towel over the cubed tofu.
- Place something heavy on top to drain.
- Allow it to rest for at least 10 minutes or accordingly.
- Bring a large pot of water to boil.
- Add the rice, boil uncovered for 30 minutes.
- Drain and return the rice to the pot.
- Cover the pot let rice simmer for 10 minutes, set aside.
- Move the pressed tofu to the lined baking sheet.
- Drizzle with the olive oil and tamari.
- Toss to combine and sprinkle the starch over the tofu toss again till evenly coated.
- Arrange the tofu in an even layer.
- Bake for 25 – 30 minutes toss halfway, until deeply golden on the edges. Set aside.
- Whisk all the ingredients together in a bowl.
- Taste and season accordingly, set aside.
- In a medium mixing bowl, combine the diced mango, bell pepper, green jalapeño, onion, lime juice, cilantro, and salt.
- Stir to combine, and set aside.
- Scoop rice top with a handful of shredded cabbage.

- Add a big scoop of mango salsa, a handful of baked tofu, a hefty drizzle of peanut sauce, and a sprinkle of chopped peanuts.
- Serve and enjoy

Halloumi tacos with pineapple salsa and aji Verde

Ingredients

- [Aji Verde](#)
- 8 small corn
- ¼ cup of extra-virgin olive oil
- [Pineapple Salsa](#)
- 8 ounces of halloumi cheese, sliced into rounds

Directions

- In a medium skillet using a medium heat, warm the tortilla through.
- Stack them together under a clean tea towel.
- In the same skillet, warm olive oil over medium heat.
- Place slices of halloumi into the hot oil.
- Cook the cheese until golden in 2 – 4 minutes.
- Flip each piece of cheese with the tongs let cook until the other side is golden 2 – 4 minutes.
- Place a few paper towels on a cutting board to absorb excess oil.
- Place cooked cheese onto the plate let cool a bit before handling.
- Slice each piece of cheese into strips.
- Place a few strips of cheese along half of your tortilla.
- Top with pineapple salsa.
- Finish each taco with a drizzle of aji Verde.
- Serve warm and enjoy.

Baked ziti with roasted vegetables

Roasted vegetables are significant in elevating this baked ziti. Prepared with mozzarella, pasta and red sauce, the baked ziti with roasted vegetables is a delicious meal.

Ingredients

- 2 cups of cottage cheese
- 1 red bell pepper
- 8 ounces of ziti, rigatoni
- 2 tablespoons of extra-virgin olive oil
- ¼ teaspoon of fine sea salt
- 1 medium head of cauliflower cut into florets
- 4 cups of marinara sauce
- ¼ cup of chopped fresh basil
- 1 medium yellow onion, wedged
- 8 ounces of grated part-skim mozzarella cheese

Directions

- Preheat your oven to 425°F.
- Line two large baking sheets with parchment paper.
- Place the cauliflower florets on one pan.
- Combine the bell peppers and onion on the other.
- Drizzle olive oil over the pans.
- Sprinkle salt over the two pans.
- Toss until the vegetables on each pan are lightly coated in oil.
- Organize the vegetables in an even layer across each pan.
- Bake for 30 – 35 minutes till the vegetables are tender and caramelized on the edges.

- Toss the veggies and swapping their rack positions halfway.
- Bring a large pot of salted water to boil.
- Cook the pasta according to package instruction.
- Drain and return to the pot.
- Add 2 cups of the marinara, the chopped basil, and ½ cup of the mozzarella, stir to combine.
- Spread 1 cup of marinara sauce inside the baker.
- Top with half of the pasta mixture, spread into an even layer.
- Sprinkle the roasted cauliflower on top.
- Dollop 1 cup of the cottage cheese over the cauliflower and ½ cup of the mozzarella.
- Top with the remaining pasta.
- Sprinkle the roasted peppers and onion on top.
- Dollop the remaining cup of ricotta and marina.
- Sprinkle the remaining cheese all over.
- Place the baking sheet on the lower oven rack to catch any drippings.
- Place the ziti, uncovered, on top of the baking sheet.
- Bake for 30 minutes
- Move to the upper rack for 2 – 5 minutes until deeply golden
- Remove the baker from the oven let cool for 10 minutes.
- Sprinkle freshly torn basil on top, slice with a knife.
- Serve and enjoy.

Thai panang curry vegetables

The recipe embraces the health power of vegetable; as such, it is fully packed with vegetables and variety of fresh flavors.

Ingredients

- Fresh Thai basil, sriracha or chili garlic sauce
- 1 tablespoon coconut oil
- 1 to 2 tablespoons panang curry paste
- 1 tablespoon tamari
- Pinch of salt
- ½ cup water
- 1 yellow, orange, sliced into strips
- 3 carrots, peeled and sliced
- 2 cloves garlic, pressed
- 1 can regular coconut milk
- 2 tablespoons peanut butter
- 1 ½ teaspoons coconut sugar
- 1 red bell pepper, sliced into strips
- 1 small white or yellow onion, chopped
- 2 teaspoons fresh lime juice

Directions

- Bring a large pot of water to boil.
- Add rice boil for 30 minutes, lower heat and simmer.
- When ready drain, return the rice to pot.
- Cover let rest for 10 minutes set aside.
- Warm a large skillet over medium heat.
- When hot, add the oil with onion and a sprinkle of salt let cook, stirring often for 5 minutes.

- Add bell peppers and carrots let cook until bell peppers can be pierced with fork 3 – 5 minutes, stirring occasionally.
- Add the garlic and curry paste
- Let cook for 1 minute, while stirring.
- Add coconut milk together with water, stir to combine.
- Simmer the mixture over medium heat.
- Adjust the heat as necessary until the peppers and carrots have softened in 5 – 10 minutes, stirring occasionally.
- Remove the pot from the heat.
- Stir in the peanut butter, sugar, tamari, and lime juice.
- Add salt and season accordingly.
- Divide rice and curry into bowls and garnish with fresh basil.
- Serve and enjoy.

Crispy baked tofu

Ingredients

- 1 block of organic extra-firm tofu
- 1 tablespoon of extra-virgin olive oil
- 1 tablespoon of tamari
- 1 tablespoon of cornstarch

Directions

- Start by preheat your oven to 400°F.
- Align a large baking sheet with parchment paper.
- Drain the tofu with you palms to gently squeeze out the water.
- Slice the tofu into thirds lengthwise.
- Stack the slabs on top of each other and slice through them lengthwise making 3 even columns.
- Slice across to make 5 even rows.
- Get a chopping board with towel.
- Arrange the tofu in an even layer on the towel cover with a heavy object to drain extra water.
- Move pressed tofu to a medium mixing bowl
- Drizzle with the olive oil and tamari.
- Toss to combine.
- Sprinkle the starch over the tofu, toss until starch is evenly coated.
- Bake for 25 – 30 minutes, toss halfway, until deeply golden on edges.
- Serve and enjoy.

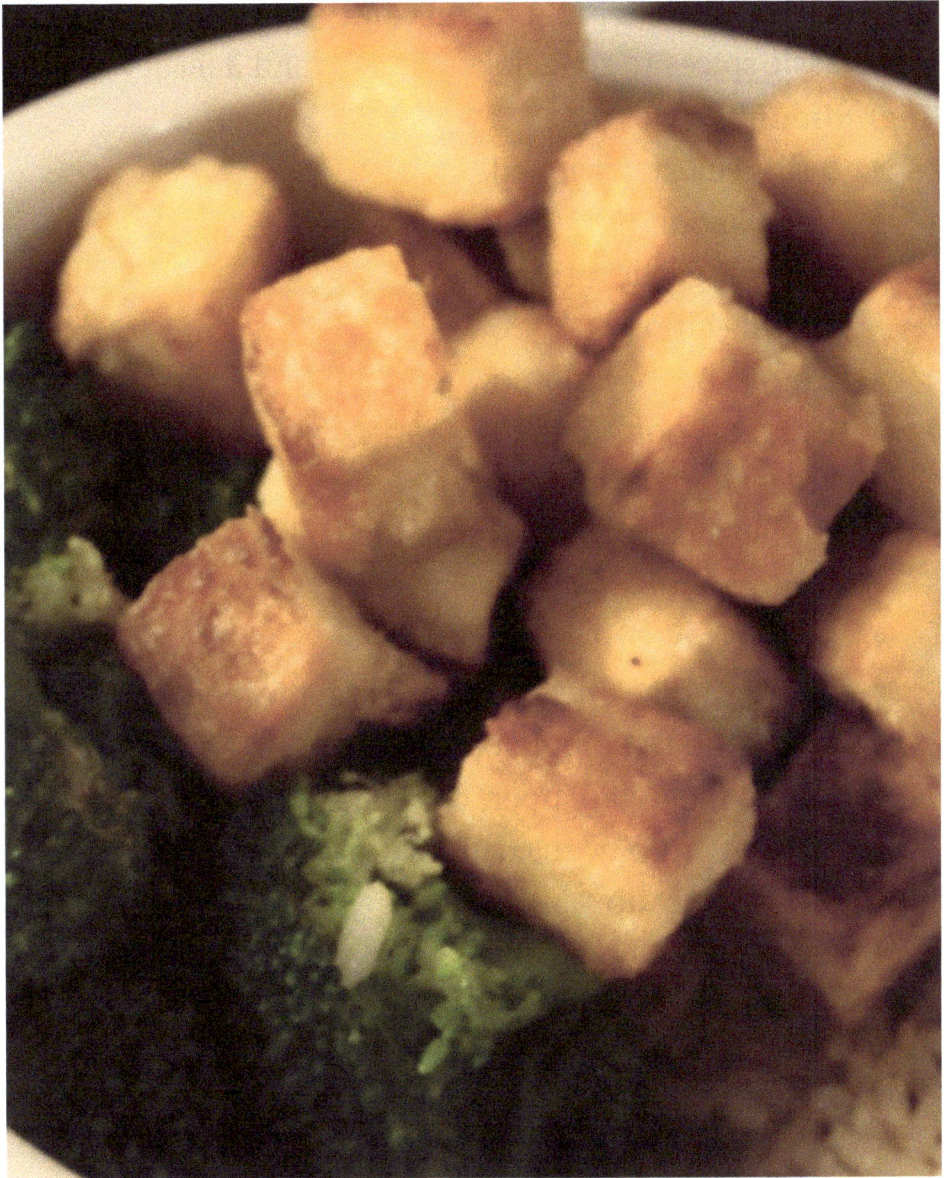

Homemade veggie chili

This recipe features smoky and complex flavors. It emerged from poultry ingredients and vegetable varieties and classic spices to spike its sweetness and delicacy.

Ingredients

- 2 ribs celery, chopped
- ½ teaspoon salt
- 4 cloves garlic, pressed
- Tortilla chips
- 2 tablespoons chili powder
- 1 ½ teaspoons smoked paprika
- 1 teaspoon dried oregano
- 2 tablespoons extra-virgin olive oil
- Sour cream
- 1 large can of diced tomatoes
- 2 cans of black beans, rinsed and drained
- 1 medium red onion, chopped
- 1 large red bell pepper, chopped
- 1 can of pinto beans, rinsed and drained
- Sliced avocado
- 2 cups of vegetable broth
- 1 bay leaf
- 2 medium carrots, chopped
- 2 tablespoons chopped fresh cilantro
- 1 to 2 teaspoons sherry vinegar
- 2 teaspoons ground cumin
- Chopped cilantro

Directions

- In a large oven warm the olive oil until shimmering without smoke over medium heat.
- Add the chopped bell pepper, onion, celery, carrot, and ¼ teaspoon of the salt stir to combine.
- Cook until the vegetables are tender, onion translucent in 7 – 10 minutes, stirring occasionally.
- Add garlic, cumin, chili powder, smoked paprika and oregano.
- Cook until fragrant, stirring constantly for 1 minute.
- Add diced tomatoes, black beans, vegetable broth, pinto beans, and bay leaf.
- Stir to combine then simmer for 30 minutes.
- Remove the chili from the heat and discard the bay leaf.
- Move 1 ½ cups of the chili to a blender, blend till smooth.
- Pour the mixture back into the pot.
- Add the chopped cilantro, stir to combine.
- Stir in the vinegar to taste.
- Add salt accordingly.
- Place in bowls serve and enjoy.

Vegetarian stuffed acorn squash

The use of quinoa filling gives this recipe a beautifully tasty flavor that you cannot possibly resist.

Ingredients

- ¼ cup raw pepitas
- ¼ cup chopped green onion
- 1 cup water
- 2 tablespoons extra-virgin olive oil
- ¼ cup chopped parsley
- 1 clove garlic minced
- 2 medium acorn squash
- ½ teaspoon fine sea salt
- 1 tablespoon lemon juice
- ¾ cup grated Parmesan cheese
- ½ cup quinoa, rinsed
- ¼ cup dried cranberries
- ½ cup crumbled goat cheese

Directions

- Preheat the oven to 400°F.
- Align a large baking sheet with parchment paper.
- Slice through the squash up to down, scoop out the seeds and stringy bits inside.
- Place the squash halves on the parchment pan.
- Drizzle 1 tablespoon of the olive oil over the squash.
- Sprinkle with ¼ teaspoon of salt.

- Rub the oil into the cut sides of the squash, face the cut sides to the pan.
- Bake until squash is easily pierced through in 30 – 45 minutes.
- In a separate medium saucepan, combine quinoa with water.
- Boil over medium-high heat, then lower heat to simmer uncovered for 12 – 18 minutes.
- Stir in the cranberries when the mixture is off heat.
- Cover let steam for 5 minutes.
- In a medium skillet, toast the pepitas over medium heat as you keep stirring frequently, until golden on the edges in 4 – 5 minutes. Keep aside.
- Put the quinoa mixture into a medium mixing bowl.
- Add the toasted garlic, pepitas, parsley, onion, lemon juice, the remaining ¼ teaspoon of salt, and 1 tablespoon of olive oil.
- Stir for even distribution.
- Taste and season accordingly.
- Add the Parmesan cheese and goat cheese stir to combine.
- Turn the cooked squash halves over.
- Divide the mixture evenly between halves a spoon.
- Return the squash to the oven let bake for 15 – 18 minutes.

- Sprinkle the stuffed squash with 1 tablespoon of chopped parsley.
- Serve warm and enjoy.

Crispy falafel

Ingredients

- ½ teaspoon of ground cumin
- ¼ cup and 1 tablespoon extra-virgin olive oil
- 1 teaspoon of fine sea salt
- ¼ teaspoon of ground cinnamon
- ½ cup of roughly chopped red onion
- ½ cup of packed fresh cilantro
- ½ teaspoon of freshly ground black pepper
- ½ cup of packed fresh parsley
- 1 cup of dried chickpeas

Directions

- Preheat oven to 375 °F.
- Pour ¼ cup of the olive oil in a large baking sheet tilt round to evenly coat.
- Combine chickpeas, onion, garlic, parsley, salt, pepper, cilantro, cumin, cinnamon, and 1 tablespoon of olive oil in a food processor. Blend for 1 minute till smooth.
- Shape the falafel into small patties, 2 inches wide, ½ inch thick.
- Place them falafel on the oiled pan.
- Bake for 25 – 30 minutes ensure to flip over to bake all sides.
- Serve and enjoy.

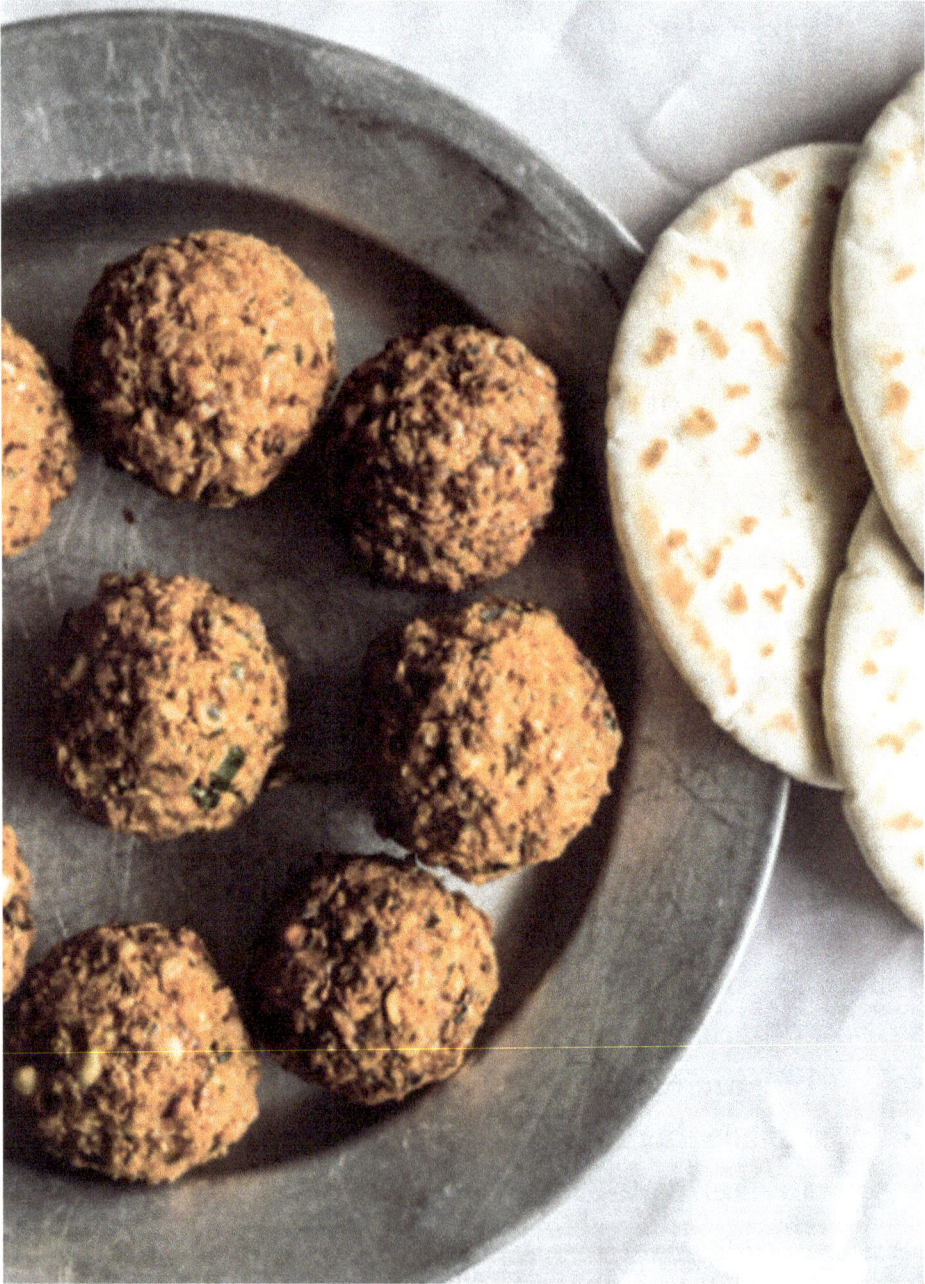

Epic vegetarian tacos

Using pickled onions, refried beans, and avocado sauce, this recipe is so delightfully delicious for a meal with meatless tacos.

Ingredients

- Creamy avocado dip
- 8 corn tortillas

- Quick-pickled onions
- Chopped fresh cilantro
- Lime wedges

- Salsa Verde
- Shredded green cabbage
- Crumbled Cotjia

- Easy refried beans

Directions

- Prepare these ingredients normally onions, avocado dip, and beans.
- In a large skillet, warm every side of the tortillas over medium temperature in batches.
- Stack the warmed tortillas on a plate and cover.
- Spread refried beans down but at the center of every tortilla.
- Top with avocado dip and onions.
- Garnish and serve.
- Enjoy.

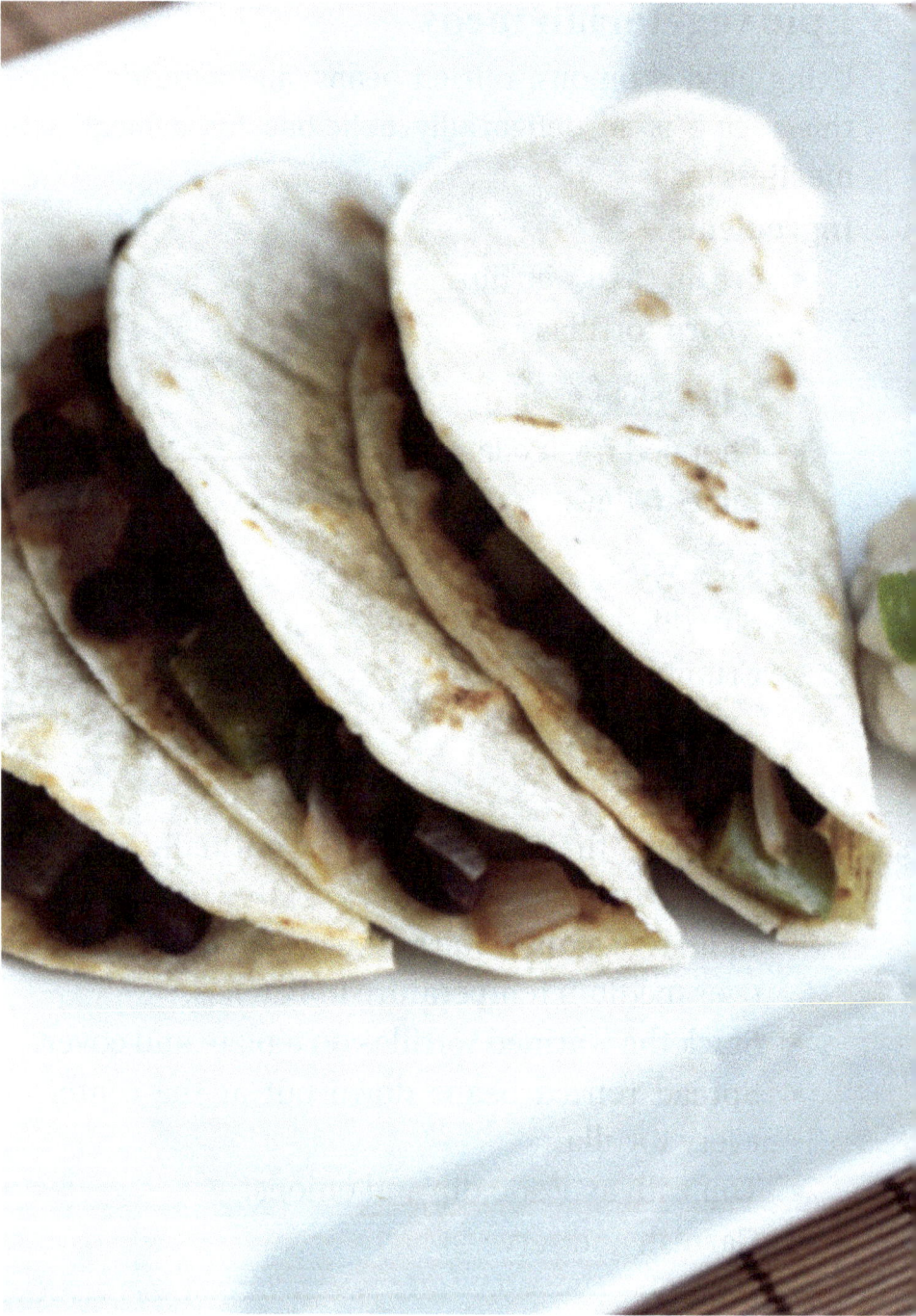

Loaded vegetables nachos

This is a quicker Mediterranean Sea diet veggies with zero percent meat. Prepared with creamy avocado sauce and cheese in 25 minutes.

Ingredients

- 1 packed cup of shredded cheddar cheese
- red bell pepper, chopped
- ⅓ cup crumbled feta cheese
- Your favorite salsa
- 1 can of pinto beans, rinsed and drained

- [Avocado dip](#)
- ⅓ cup chopped green onions
- 1 packed cup of shredded Monterey Jack cheese
- 2 radishes, chopped
- Pickled jalapeños
- 2 tablespoons chopped cilantro

Directions

- Begin by preheating your oven to 400°F.
- Align a baking sheet with parchment paper.
- Place handfuls of chips on the baking sheet distributed evenly.
- Sprinkle the prepared pan of chips evenly with the beans and so the shredded cheese, crumbled feta, bell pepper, and pickled jalapeños.
- Bake until the cheese is melted in 9 – 13 minutes.
- When ready, remove, set aside.
- Drizzle the nachos with avocado sauce.

- Sprinkle the nachos with radish, onion, and cilantro.
- Serve soon enough and enjoy when still warm.

Pinto posole

The vegetarian type pinto posole features beans instead of pork.

This recipe is spicy, flavorful and delicious to light up your taste buds.

Ingredients

- ½ teaspoon fine sea salt
- 2 tablespoons extra-virgin olive oil
- 1 lime, halved
- 1 tablespoon ground cumin
- ½ cup of tomato paste
- 1 bay leaf
- 2 cups water
- 3 cans of pinto beans, rinsed and drained
- 2 to 4 guajillo chili peppers
- 1 can of hominy, rinsed and drained
- 32 ounces of vegetable broth
- 4 cloves garlic, pressed or minced
- 1 large white onion, finely chopped
- ¼ cup chopped cilantro

Directions

- Heat your oven over a medium heat until it evaporates.
- Toast the chili press flat with a spatula briefly till fragrant flip over repeat.
- In the same pot, warm the olive oil until shimmering without smoke.

- Add the onion and a pinch of salt.
- Cook while stirring frequently, until onions turn translucent in 5 minutes.
- Add the garlic together with cumin let cook until fragrant in 1 minute.
- Add the tomato paste cook for 1 minute, keep stirring.
- Add toasted chili peppers, hominy, bay leaf, vegetable broth, beans, and water to the pot.
- Stir in salt and raise the heat to medium.
- Simmer regulate the heat for 25 minutes.
- Discard the chili peppers and bay leaf..
- Stir the cilantro and juice of lime into the soup.
- Taste and season accordingly.
- Garnish with lime wedges.
- Serve and enjoy.

Real stovetop mac and cheese

Ingredients

- Tiny pinch of cayenne pepper
- ⅓ cup of heavy cream
- 1 ⅓ packed cups of sharp cheddar cheese
- 8 ounces of regular macaroni noodles
- ⅛ teaspoon of onion powder
- ½ teaspoon of mustard powder
- 2 teaspoons of salt
- ⅛ teaspoon of garlic powder

Directions

- Bring water to boil in a medium pot.
- Add noodles and salt.
- Let cook according to package Directions.
- Drain the pasta let stay in the colander.
- Return the same pot heat.
- Add cream let boil time for 1 minute.
- Add cheese with spices when the timer is up, stir till cheese has melted.
- Add boiled pasta, stir to coated in cheese sauce.
- Remove the pot from the heat source.
- Taste and season accordingly.
- Best served and enjoyed immediately.

Super simple marinara sauce

With only 5 core ingredients, this marinara sauce is quite simple to make yet very delicious. Here, there is no struggle in chopping this and that because it is not needed.

Ingredients

- Salt
- 1 medium yellow onion
- 2 large cloves garlic left whole
- Pinch of red pepper flakes
- 1 large can of whole peeled tomatoes
- 1 teaspoon of dried oregano
- 2 tablespoons of extra-virgin olive oil

Directions

- Combine tomatoes, garlic cloves, olive oil, halved onion, oregano and red pepper flakes in a medium saucepan.
- Simmer over low heat for 45 minutes.
- Stir occasionally, crush tomatoes with the back of a spoon.
- Take off the pot from heat source, throw the onion.
- Stir smashed garlic into the sauce.
- Add salt season to taste.
- Serve warm and enjoy.
- Leftover can be refrigerated for later consumption.

Hearty spaghetti with lentils and marinara

This is a recipe for typical whole meal with lentils, spaghetti, variety of vegetables, and marinara sauce for lunch or dinner. It comes delightfully delicious in only 35 minutes. You can surely wait for that times. Don't you?

Ingredients

- 8 ounces of whole-grain pasta
- 1 bay leaf
- 2 cups of marinara sauce
- 1 large garlic clove, left whole
- ¼ teaspoon of salt
- ½ cup of dry lentils
- 2 cups of vegetable broth

Directions

- In a small saucepan, combine the bay leaf, garlic, lentils, salt, and broth.
- Simmer over medium-high heat for 20 – 35 minutes till the lentils have cooked through.
- Drain the lentils, throw away bay leaf and garlic. Keep uncovered.
- Boil salted water in a large saucepan.
- Place in the pasta, cook according to package instruction.
- Drain, return to the pot keep.
- Stir the marinara into the lentils, warm over medium heat.

- Divide pasta into bowls.
- Top with warm marinara and lentils.
- Serve and enjoy warm.

Creamy pumpkin marinara

In a period of 25 minutes, this recipe will be read. It readily tastes like fall with comfort just like mac with cheese stuffed with variety of vegetables; of course it is a Mediterranean Sea diet, do not expect anything less vegetarian,

Ingredients

- Finely grated Parmesan and chopped parsley
- 1 red bell pepper, chopped
- ½ teaspoon of dried oregano
- 2 teaspoons of balsamic vinegar
- ¼ teaspoon of dried tarragon
- ¼ teaspoon of ground cinnamon
- 1 can of diced tomatoes
- 1 can of pumpkin purée
- ½ teaspoon of salt, divided
- 2 tablespoons of butter
- 2 cloves garlic, minced
- 2 tablespoons of extra-virgin olive oil
- 1 yellow onion, chopped
- Freshly ground black pepper

Directions

- In a large skillet, warm olive oil over medium heat.
- Let shimmer without smoke.
- Add onion, bell pepper and salt.
- Let cook while stirring frequently, till onions and pepper are tender in 8 minutes.

- Add garlic, tarragon, oregano, and cinnamon let cook for 1 minute.
- Introduce tomatoes let cook for 1 minute.
- Stir in the pumpkin purée, stir to combine.
- Simmering for 5 minutes over low heat.
- Move the mixture to a blender.
- Add 1 butter together with the vinegar.
- Blend until very smooth.
- Season with ground black pepper and salt.
- Stir in the warm pasta.
- Serve with grated Parmesan and chopped parsley.
- Enjoy

Steel cut oat risotto with butternut squash and kale

Ingredients

- 1 ½ cups of Quaker steel-cut oats
- 1 teaspoon salt
- 2 packed cups chopped kale
- ½ cup dry white wine
- Freshly ground black pepper
- 6 cups water
- 1 small butternut squash
- 1 medium red onion, chopped
- ¾ cup of freshly grated Parmesan cheese
- 2 tablespoons butter
- 2 tablespoons extra-virgin olive oil
- 1 tablespoon lemon juice
- Pinch of red pepper flakes
- 4 cloves garlic or minced

Directions

- Warm olive oil until shimmering without smoke in a medium sized oven.
- Add butternut, onion, salt, and red pepper flakes.
- Let cook until the onion is translucent in 8 – 10 minutes.
- Add garlic together with oats, kale cook to combine in 2 minutes while stirring.
- Add the wine and scape up with silicone spatula till brown bits form at the bottom.

- Continue to cook for more 2 minutes keep stirring.
- Add water and remaining salt.
- Increased the heat to high let it boil.
- Lower the heat to allow simmering for 20 – 30 minutes. Ensure the bottom does not scorch
- Stir in the butter, Parmesan, lemon juice and black pepper.
- Let rest for 5 minutes.
- Divide in bowls, serve and enjoy.

Buddha bowl

- This is another versatile recipe with rice and variety of fresh vegetables.
- **Ingredients**
- Flaky sea salt
- 1 to 2 tablespoons reduced-sodium tamari or soy sauce
- 4 cups chopped red cabbage
- Sesame seeds
- 2 ripe avocados, halved, pitted sliced into strips
- Toasted sesame oil
- 1 ½ cups frozen shelled edamame
- 1 small cucumber, thinly sliced

- Carrot ginger dressing
- 1 ¼ cups short-grain brown rice
- Thinly sliced green onion
- 1 ½ cups trimmed and roughly chopped snap peas
- Lime wedges

Directions

- Bring a large pot of water to boil.
- Add the rice let boil for 25 minutes.
- Add edamame continue to cook for 3 more minutes.
- Add snap peas cook for more 2 minutes.
- Drain excess water when ready.
- Add veggies and return to the pot.

- Season with tamari, stir to combine.
- Divide mixture and raw veggies into 4 bowls.
- Assemble the cucumber slices along the edge of the bowl.
- Drizzle lightly with carrot ginger dressing.
- Top with sliced green onion.
- Place 2 wedges in each bowl.
- Divide the avocado into the bowls, then drizzle with sesame oil, sprinkle with sesame seeds and sea salt.
- Serve and enjoy immediately.

Quick dal makhani

The quick dal makhani is loaded with variety of flavors, and naturally, it is a rich creamy recipe quick to make in 45 minutes.

Ingredients

- 1 medium yellow onion, chopped
- 1 bay leaf
- 1 can of kidney beans
- 1 tablespoon minced fresh ginger
- Chopped fresh cilantro
- 1 jalapeño pepper

- ½ teaspoon of frontier co-op ground cumin
- 2 tablespoons avocado oil
- ½ teaspoon salt
- Freshly ground black pepper
- 1 can of diced tomatoes
- 1 cup of black lentils
- 3 cloves garlic, minced

- ½ teaspoon of frontier co-op ground coriander
- 5 cups of water
- 1 ½ teaspoons of garam masala
- 1 tablespoon lime juice

Directions

- In a large pot, warm oil until shimmering without smoke over medium heat.

- Add ginger, onion, garlic, and jalapeño let cook to softened in 4 – 6 minutes. Keep stirring.
- Stir in the cumin, garam masala, coriander and salt.
- Season with black pepper.
- Cook for 1 minute.
- Add tomatoes cook for 1 minute.
- Add the lentils together with the kidney beans, water, and bay leaf.
- Increase the heat to medium-high boil for 20 minutes, lower the heat to simmer for 15 minutes.
- Move 2 cups of the mixture to a blender.
- Blend until smooth.
- Move the mixture to the pot, stir to combine.
- Add lime juice and season to taste with salt and pepper.
- Serve in bowls, with chopped cilantro and a lime wedge on top.
- Serve with rice and enjoy.

Vegetable paella

This vegetable is loaded with smoky rice and savory making it perfect for dinner parties. It is gluten free; thus vegetarian and fit for a Mediterranean Sea diet.

Ingredients

- 1 ½ teaspoons fine sea salt
- 2 tablespoons of lemon juice
- 2 red bell peppers, stemmed, seeded and sliced
- 6 garlic cloves, minced.
- 1 can of diced tomatoes
- ½ cup of frozen peas
- 2 cups of brown rice
- 1 can of chickpeas
- ¼ cup of chopped fresh parsley
- 3 cups of vegetable broth
- ⅓ cup dry white wine
- ½ teaspoon saffron threads
- 1 can of quartered artichokes
- 2 teaspoons smoked paprika
- ½ cup of Kalamata olives
- 1 medium yellow onion.
- 3 tablespoons extra-virgin olive oil
- Freshly ground black pepper.

Directions

- Preheat your oven to 350°F.
- Heat 2 tablespoons of oil in your over medium heat to shimmer without smoke.

- Add onion and a pinch of salt.
- Let cook until the onions are tender in 5 minutes.
- Carefully, stir in garlic and paprika let cook until fragrant in 30 seconds.
- Stir in tomatoes let cook until the mixture darkens somehow in 2 minutes.
- Stir in the rice and cook until the grains are well coated in 1 minute.
- Add the chickpeas, wine, broth, saffron, and 1 teaspoon salt.
- Increase the heat to medium let boil, stirring occasionally.
- Cover the pot, transfer to lower rack, let bake, till liquid is fully absorbed in 30 – 35 minutes.
- Align a large baking sheet with parchment paper.
- Combine the artichoke, chopped olives, peppers, bit of olive oil, salt, and ground black pepper, toss briefly.
- Spread the mixture across the pan.
- Roast the vegetables on the upper rack contents are tender in 40 - 45 minutes.
- Remove from oven, add parsley with lemon juice, toss.
- Season with salt and pepper. Keep.
- Sprinkle peas and roasted vegetables over baked rice.
- Cover to settle paella for 5 minutes.
- Serve and enjoy.

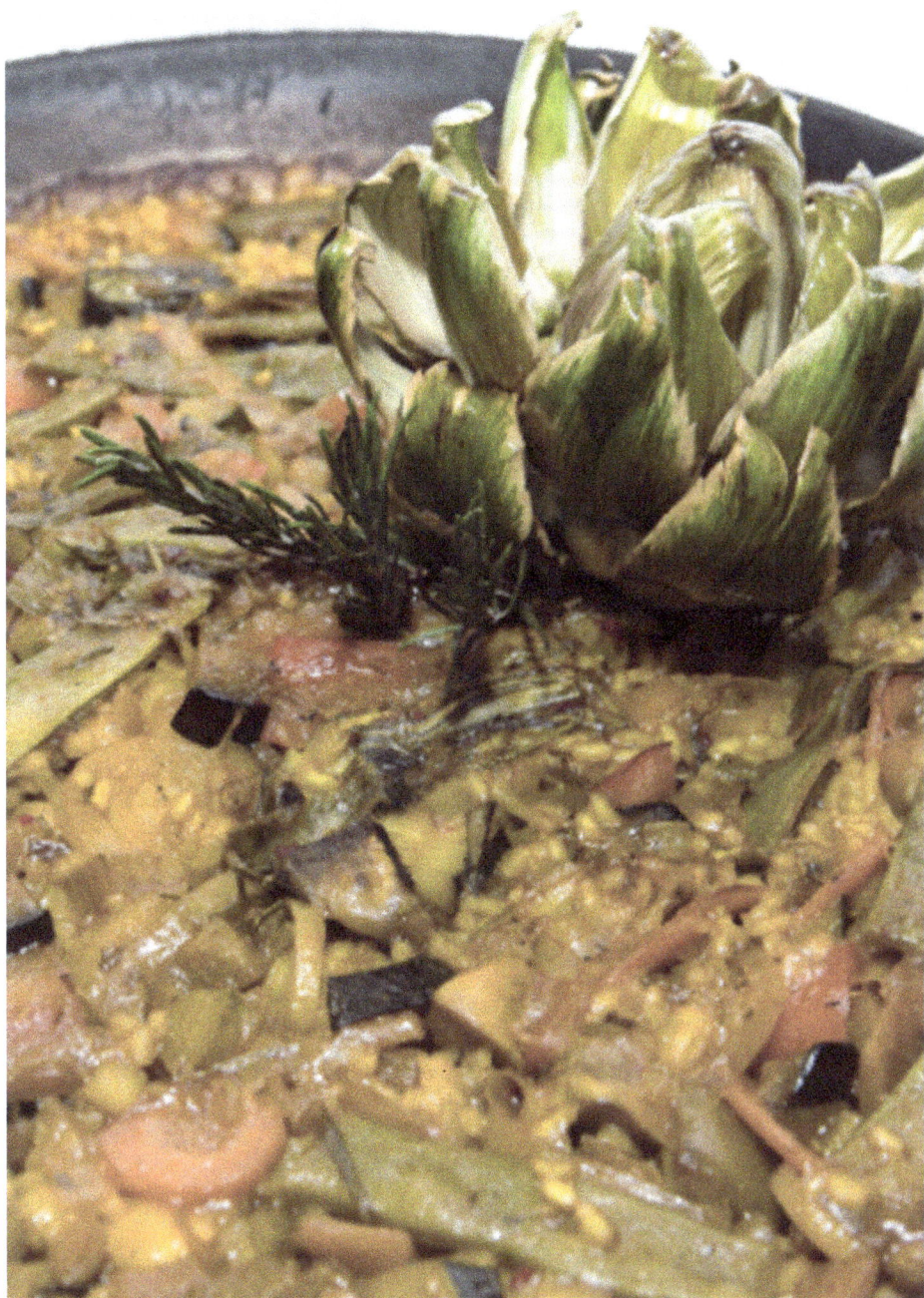

Chilaquiles Verde with baked tortilla chips

This recipe is Mexican by genesis fantastic for breakfast, lunch and dinner prepared with tortilla chips.

Ingredients

- 2 tablespoons of chopped cilantro
- ⅓ cup of crumbled Cotjia
- 2 teaspoons of extra-virgin olive oil
- 3 cups of salsa Verde
- 16 corn tortillas

- 4 fried eggs
- 1 avocado
- ½ teaspoon of sea salt
- 3 tablespoons of chopped red onion or green onion
- 2 tablespoons of extra-virgin olive oil
- 2 tablespoons of chopped fresh cilantro

Directions

- Preheat your oven to 400°F.
- Align two large baking sheets with parchment paper.
- Brush the tortilla lightly with oil.
- Stack and slice them into 8 wedges for all.
- Arrange them evenly across the pans.
- Sprinkle salt over all the pans.

- Bake, swapping the pans on their racks every 5 minutes, until the chips are curling up at the edges in 10 minutes.
- Warm 2 teaspoons of the olive oil in a large skillet over medium heat.
- Add the salsa Verde once the pan is hot enough.
- Lower the heat to simmer, then remove the skillet from the heat.
- Stir in the tortilla chips with cilantro to coated all chips
- Cover and let the rest until soft in 2 – 5 minutes.
- Add the toppings.
- Serve and enjoy.

Vegan mac and cheese

Ingredients

- 1 head of broccoli
- 3 teaspoons of apple cider vinegar
- 1 small yellow onion
- ½ teaspoon of garlic powder
- ½ teaspoon of onion powder
- ½ teaspoon of dry mustard powder

- Small pinch of red pepper flakes
- 3 cloves garlic, minced
- ⅔ cup of raw cashews
- 1 ½ tablespoons of avocado oil
- 8 ounces of whole-grain macaroni elbows
- 1 cup of water
- 1 cup of peeled and grated russet potato
- ½ teaspoon of salt
- ¼ cup of yeast

Directions

- Boil salted water in a large pot. Place in the pasta and cook according to package instruction.
- Drain, and transfer to a large serving bowl when not completely ready.
- Warm oil over medium heat.
- Add onion and a pinch of salt let cook, until the onion translucent in 5 minutes.
- Add the grated potato, garlic powder, garlic, mustard powder, onion powder, salt and red

pepper flakes stir to combine and cook for 1 minute.

- Add cashews with water, stir to combine.
- Simmer over reduced heat, stirring frequently for 5 – 8 minutes.
- Pour mixture into a blender together with yeast and vinegar. Blend. For 2 minutes.
- Taste and blend accordingly.
- Transfer the sauce into the bowl of pasta. Stir to combine.
- Serve soon enough and enjoy.

Almond sesame soda noodles with quick-pickled veggies

Ingredients

- 1 large cucumber
- 2 teaspoons of salt, divided
- 1 tablespoon sesame seeds
- ½ cup of unsalted almond butter
- Sriracha
- 1 small garlic clove, minced
- ¼ cup of freshly squeezed lime juice
- 2 tablespoons of tamari
- 8 ounces of soba noodles
- 2 teaspoons of raw honey
- 1 bunch of radishes
- 2 teaspoons toasted sesame oil
- ¼ cup water
- ¼ cup of rice vinegar
- 2 large zucchini

Directions

- Start by cooking the noodles as per the package instruction, set aside after draining.
- Combine cucumber with vinegar, radishes, and salt, let marinate for 10 minutes keep tossing.
- In a smaller mixing bowl, combine garlic, almond butter, lime juice, honey, tamari, sesame oil and salt whisk to until blended. Place little water blend again briefly as required.

- Place the sauce into the mixing bowl together with the soba noodles.
- Add zucchini noodles toss to coated.
- Put in serving dishes, top with quick-pickled veggies.
- Garnish with sesame seeds.
- Serve at room temperature.
- Enjoy.

Broccolini almond pizza

Red sauce and mozzarella with blanched broccolini makes the perfect delicious pizza best for breakfast, lunch and dinner in less than 40 minutes.

Ingredients

- Red pepper flakes
- ¼ cup of sliced almonds

- ⅔ cup pizza sauce
- ½ cup of crumbled feta
- 1 batch easy whole wheat
- ½ pound of broccolini
- 1 teaspoon of extra-virgin olive oil
- 2 cups shredded low-moisture mozzarella cheese

Directions

- Preheat your oven to 500°F.
- Spread marinara sauce evenly over the pizza.
- Pour the mozzarella, feta and almonds over the pizza.
- Boil water in a saucepan. Trim the broccolini.
- Toss in the broccolini, let boil for 1 minute.
- Drain and pat dry.
- Then, toss again with 1 teaspoon of olive oil to coat lightly.
- Assemble the broccolini over the pizza.
- Sprinkle the almonds on top.
- Bake pizza on the top rack until golden in 12 minutes.

- Transfer to a cutting board
- Sprinkle with red pepper flakes.
- Slice, serve and enjoy.

Hummus quesadillas

Unlike with cheese, this quesadilla is typically prepared with hummus delicious enough to keep you hooked the whole day. it is gluten and dairy free vegan healthy recipe.

Ingredients

- One 8-inch whole grain tortilla
- ⅓ cup hummus
- Fillings of your choice
- Extra-virgin olive oil

Directions

- Begin by spreading hummus over the tortilla.
- Lightly cover one-half of the tortilla with fillings.
- Fold the blank half over. Make as needed.
- Warm a medium skillet over medium heat.
- Place folded quesadilla(s) in the pan.
- Warm lower sides briefly. Brush with olive oil, let cook in the pan for 2 minutes. Repeat this step for the other side. Continue to cook until all sides turn golden.
- Transfer to a cutting board let rest briefly.
- Slice into 3 wedges.
- Serve and enjoy.

Lentil baked ziti

Ingredients

- Basil leaves
- 2 cloves garlic, minced
- 1 ¼ cups of regular brown lentils
- 3 cups of water
- ¼ teaspoon of salt
- Freshly ground black pepper
- Pinch of red pepper flakes
- 1 red onion
- 23.5 ounces of [Marinara](#)
- 1 tablespoon of olive oil
- 8 ounces of grated mozzarella cheese
- 1 cup cottage cheese
- 12 ounces of whole grain ziti

Directions

- Warm olive oil until shimmering without smoke in a large saucepan.
- Add onion and salt cook until onions turn translucent in 5 minutes
- Add garlic let cook for 30 seconds or until fragrant.
- Add lentils with water, stir to combine.
- Increase the heat to high, then lower after 25 minutes, let simmer over low heat for 15 minutes.
- Drain out excess water. Set aside.
- Preheat your oven to 350°F.

- Place salted water to boil in a large saucepan. Place the pasta to cook as instructed on the package.
- Drain excess water return to the saucepan.
- Add the lentils to the pasta.
- Add cheese, leave some for later.
- Season to taste with salt and freshly ground black pepper.
- Pour to the baking dish evenly spread the sauce to coat.
- Pour the lentil together with pasta into the baker, spread. Dollop cheese over the mixture.
- Drizzle the balance over the dish.
- Cover the baker tightly. Bake for 30 minutes.
- Continue baking when uncovered at higher heat until golden.
- Remove the baker from the oven let it cool for 10 minutes.
- Sprinkle with basil.
- Serve and enjoy.

Spring veggie stir fry

This meal gets ready only in 20 minutes served with rice and any protein source.

Ingredients

- 2 teaspoons of arrowroot starch
- 3 medium carrots
- 1 tablespoon of grated fresh ginger
- ½ bunch of thin asparagus
- Pinch of salt
- 1 large clove garlic minced
- ½ teaspoon of crushed red pepper
- 1 tablespoon of coconut oil
- ¼ cup of Soy Sauce
- 2 tablespoons of Wildflower Honey
- 1 small red onion

Directions

- Combine soy sauce, cornstarch, honey, garlic, ginger, and red pepper flakes. Whisk until blended.
- Warm oil over medium temperature until shimmering without smoke.
- Add onion together with carrots and salt.
- Increase the heat to high cook, stirring frequently to soften onions in 5 minutes.
- Add asparagus let cook for 3 minutes or until carrots begin to caramelize on the edges.

- Pour in the prepared sauce and cook for 1 minute or until thick.
- Serve and enjoy.

Sweet potato and black bean tacos

Beans could not be any more delicious with avocado pepitas dip. The recipe takes only 30 minutes to prepare this vegan meal for lunch or dinner or even breakfast.

Ingredients
- Olive oil
- Salt
- Ground cumin
- Crumbled feta
- 2 cans of black beans
- Water
- 2 avocado pitted
- 1 cup of lightly packed fresh cilantro
- 2 pounds of sweet potatoes
- ½ cup pepitas
- 1 small jalapeño
- Ground black pepper
- 2 cloves garlic
- ¼ teaspoon of cayenne pepper
- 1 teaspoon of cherry vinegar
- 2 tablespoons lime juice
- 1 yellow onion
- 10 small corn tortillas
- ¼ teaspoon of chili powder

Directions
- Preheat the oven to 425°F.
- Align a large baking sheet with parchment paper.

- Toss potatoes with olive oil, cayenne pepper, and salt.
- Organize in a single layer bake for 30 – 40 minutes toss halfway, until tender.
- Warm the olive oil in a large saucepan over medium heat.
- Add onions sprinkled with salt let cook for 5 – 8 minutes until onions turn translucent.
- Add cumin together with the chili powder pour beans and water after 1 minute. Simmer over low heat covered.
- Smash some of the beans then stir in the vinegar, season with salt and pepper.
- Toast pepitas in a skillet over medium heat for 5 minutes. Transfer to a bowl, set aside.
- Place avocado flesh into a food processor with jalapeño, cilantro, garlic, lime juice, water and salt. Blend until smooth.
- Add the pepitas, process till they are chopped.
- Taste and season accordingly. Keep in a small bowl.
- Warm the tortillas.
- Spread black beans down the middle of each tortilla.
- Top with bit of sweet potatoes and avocado dip.
- Garnish with feta and pepitas.
- Serve and enjoy.

Vegan BLT sandwich

This tasty vegan sandwich is prepared with variety of vegetable; tomatoes, avocado, and coconut bacon. It is quite classic on the Mediterranean Sea diet menu for lunch and dinner in 12 minutes.

Ingredients

- 1 medium ripe avocado
- Salt
- Freshly ground black pepper
- Several small leaves of romaine

- ¼ cup of [coconut bacon](#)
- 1 medium ripe red tomato
- 2 slices of eureka

Instruction

- Toast bread to your liking.
- Scoop the avocado flesh into a bowl with a pinch of salt.
- Mash the avocado with fork, till smooth.
- Spread the bread with avocado.
- Spread coconut bacon heavily on one piece of toast.
- Press into the avocado to stick.
- Slice the tomato into slices.
- Top the bacon-covered toast with slices of tomato.
- Sprinkle with black pepper.
- Top tomato with lettuce and the other bread on top, avocado side down.

- Enjoy the bites.

Vegan spaghetti alla puttanesca

If you are seeking for an ultimate super fresh taste, then seek no more, vegan spaghetti alla puttanesca prepared with pantry staple is a delicious vegan meal.

Ingredients

- 1 tablespoon of caper brine
- 3 cloves garlic, minced
- ½ cup chopped parsley leaves
- 1 tablespoon of olive oil
- 8 ounces of whole grain spaghetti
- ⅓ cup of chopped Kalamata olives
- Freshly ground black pepper
- ¼ teaspoon of red pepper flakes
- 1 large can of chunky tomato sauce
- ⅓ cup of capers
- Salt
- 1 tablespoon of Kalamata olive brine

Directions

- Combine tomato sauce, olive bring, capers, olives, caper brine, garlic, and red pepper flakes in a saucepan.
- Cook over high heat, then reduce heat to simmer, in 20 minute, keep stirring frequently.
- Remove from heat, stir in olive oil and chopped parsley season with ground black pepper and salt.
- As the sauce is cooking, place salted water in a large saucepan, cook as directed on the package.

- Drain and return it to the pot.
- Pour sauce over the pasta, stir gently to combine.
- Place into bowls, top each bowl with a light sprinkle of parsley.
- Serve immediately and enjoy.

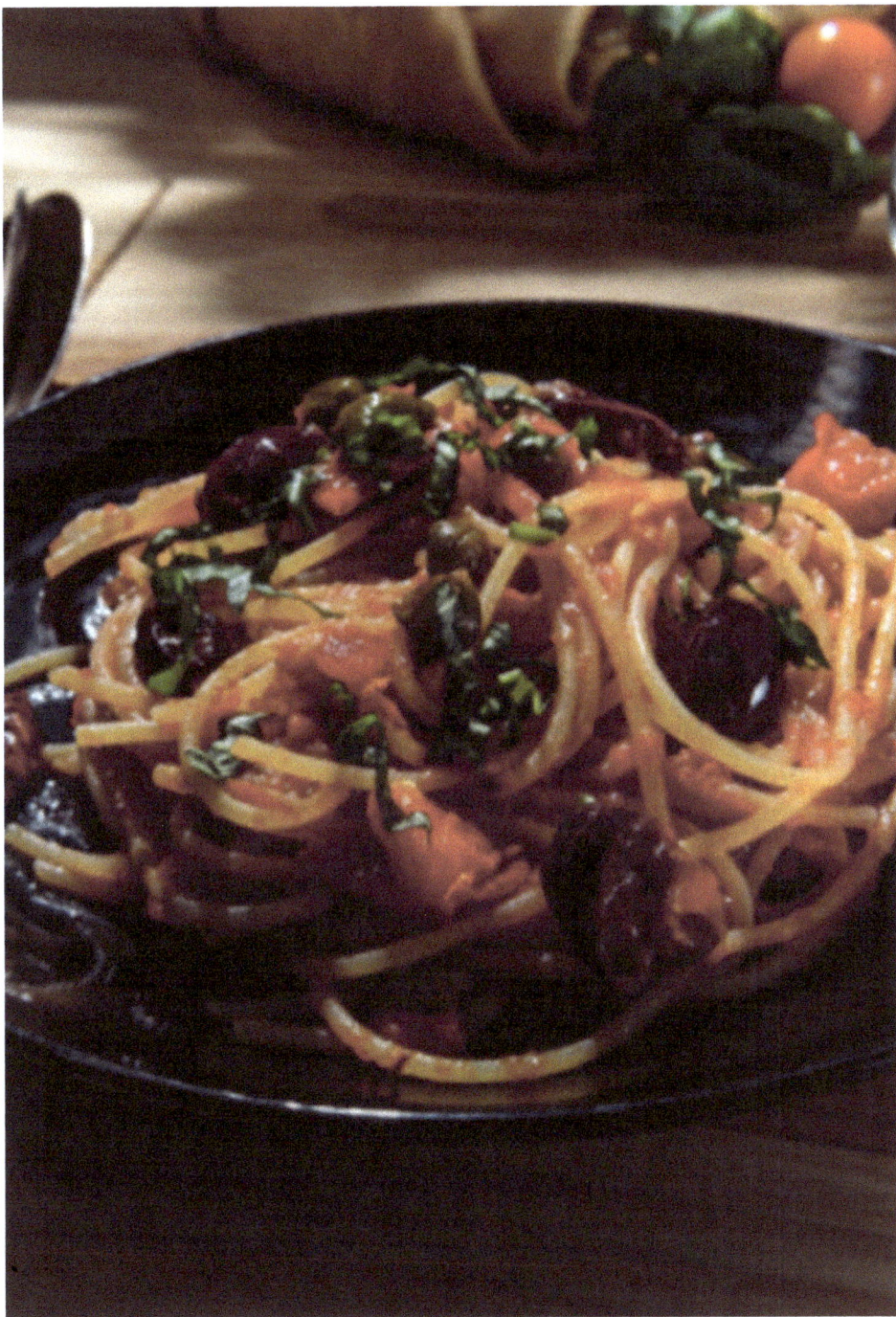

Zucchini noodles with basil pumpkin

Ingredients

- ½ cup of pepitas
- Salt
- 1 garlic clove
- 2 cups of packed fresh basil leaves
- ⅓ cup of olive oil
- 2 teaspoons of red wine vinegar
- Pinch of red pepper flakes
- 3 large zucchini
- ½ small yellow onion
- Fresh basil leaves
- 1 pint of cherry tomatoes

Instruction

- In a food processor, combine garlic, onion, toasted pepitas, basil, olive oil, vinegar and red pepper flakes.
- Blend until smooth, season with salt.
- Toss zucchini with pesto until coated, season with salt.
- Transfer to a large platter.
- Sprinkle with the cherry tomatoes.
- Serve and enjoy.

Better broccoli casserole

This recipe takes another twist of roasted broccoli, with creamy quinoa and garlicky whole grain bread crumbs along with cheddar cheese. This undeniably healthy recipe is an amazing choice for breakfast or dinner.

Ingredients

- 1 slice of whole wheat bread
- 1 clove garlic minced
- 2 cups of vegetable broth or water
- Freshly ground black pepper
- ¾ teaspoon of salt
- ¼ teaspoon of red pepper flakes
- 1 cup of quinoa
- 8 ounces of freshly grated cheddar cheese
- 1 cup of low-fat milk
- 2 tablespoons of olive oil
- ½ tablespoon of butter
- 16 ounces of broccoli florets

Directions

- Preheat oven to 400 °F.
- Line a large baking sheet with parchment paper
- Boil water in a medium sized saucepan.
- Add quinoa, reduce heat to let simmer uncovered for 18 – 20 minutes.
- Remove and steam for 10 minutes when covered.
- Slice large broccoli to small pieces.

- Move to baking sheet, toss with olive oil, until coated.
- Arrange in a single layer then Sprinkle with salt.
- Bake for 20 minutes, until tender.
- Toss bread and place in a food processor. Process until broken into crumbs.
- Melt butter in a small pan over medium heat.
- Add garlic cook until fragrant.
- Add the bread crumbs cook for 3 minutes keep aside.
- Over low heat add salt, pepper and red pepper flakes to the pot of quinoa make sure to stir to combine.
- Add cheese to the pot with milk stir to blend.
- Pour mixture in a dish, top with roasted broccoli. Stir.
- Sprinkle the casserole with cheese and breadcrumbs on top.
- Bake while uncovered for 25 minutes.
- Cool, serve and enjoy.

Spinach pasta with roasted broccoli and bell pepper

The vegetables are tossed with flavorful balsamic sauce and massively loaded with vegetables; spinach pasta. It is gluten free and vegan for a complete meal.

Ingredients

- Freshly ground black pepper
- 1 red bell pepper
- 2 tablespoons of balsamic vinegar
- Salt
- 1 shallot bulb.
- ¼ teaspoon of red pepper flakes
- 2 cloves garlic, pressed or minced
- 1 large bunch of broccoli
- 12 ounces of baby spinach
- 8 ounces of spaghetti
- 4 tablespoon of olive oil
- 1 tablespoon of lemon juice

Directions

- Preheat your oven to 400°F.
- Move broccoli florets with bell pepper to the baking sheet.
- Drizzle with olive oil, toss to coated in oil.
- Sprinkle with salt, then organize the vegetables in an even layer, bake until the broccoli is tender in 25 minutes.
- Place salted water in a large pot, boil.

- Cook past as directed on the package.
- Drain and reserve some pasta water.
- Get large pan, sauté over medium heat, place olive oil to shimmer.
- Add shallot, salt and red pepper flakes cook for 5 minutes till shallots are translucent.
- Add garlic let cook 20 seconds and spinach to wilt, repeat for all spinach.
- Pour in balsamic vinegar take pot off heat source.
- Combine roasted vegetables with cooked pasta and spinach mixture.
- Add lemon juice, olive oil.
- Drizzle with pasta cooking water, toss.
- Season to taste with salt and freshly ground black pepper.
- Serve and enjoy.

Spaghetti squash burrito bowls

Ingredients

- Salt
- Freshly ground black pepper
- 2 cups purple cabbage
- Fresh lime juice
- 1 can of black beans.
- 1 red bell pepper, chopped
- 2 tablespoons olive oil
- Fresh cilantro
- ¾ cup of mild salsa Verde
- 1 medium garlic clove
- 2 medium spaghetti squash
- 1 ripe avocado, diced
- ⅓ cup chopped green onions

Directions

- Preheat the oven to 400°F.
- Prepare a large baking sheet with parchment paper.
- Drizzle spaghetti squash with olive oil, rub all over each of the halves.
- Sprinkle the insides of the squash with freshly ground black pepper, salt.
- Roast for 45 minutes, until easily pierced through.
- In a medium mixing bowl, combine black beans, cabbage, bell pepper, cilantro, green onion, olive

oil, lime juice, and salt. Toss. Keep aside as it marinates.

- In a separate bowl of a blender, combine cilantro, salsa Verde, avocado, lime juice, and garlic. Blend until smooth.
- Divide the slaw into spaghetti squash
- Add avocado salsa Verde.
- Sprinkle again with pepper and cilantro.
- Serve and enjoy.

Pasta primavera

This pasta features a bunch of healthy roasted Mediterranean vegetables for a powerful dish. Season it with thyme and oregano for a tastier recipe.

Ingredients

- 8 oz.. of grape tomatoes halved
- 3 carrots peeled and cut into short sticks
- Black pepper
- 1 red bell pepper cored and sliced into thin sticks
- ½ cup parmesan cheese more to your liking
- Zest of 1 large lemon
- 1 yellow or orange bell pepper cored and sliced
- 1 red onion halved and sliced
- 3 large garlic cloves minced
- 1 tablespoons of dried oregano more for later
- 2 zucchini halved length-wise and sliced
- 1 ½ teaspoon of fresh thyme more for later
- Kosher salt

- Extra virgin olive oil
- 2 yellow squash halved length-wise and sliced
- 12 ounces of short pasta

Directions

- Heat your oven to 450°F.
- Place the vegetables in a large mixing bowl at once.
- Add garlic, oregano, and thyme.

- Season with a pinch of kosher salt and black pepper.
- Drizzle a good amount of extra virgin olive oil. Toss.
- Move the vegetables to a large sheet pan.
- Spread them out well.
- Then, roast in heated oven for 20 minutes.
- Cook pasta in salted boiling water as per the Directions on the package.
- Drain and excess water reserving some for later.
- Move pasta to a large bowl.
- Season with salt and pepper and little oregano and fresh thyme.
- Place in the vegetables.
- Now, add the tomatoes together with the lemon zest.
- Add a bit of the reserved pasta cooking water with a bit of extra virgin olive oil. Toss.
- Sprinkle with parmesan cheese.
- Serve and enjoy immediately.

Lemon broccoli pesto pasta

Prepared with a splash of lemon, this lemon pesto pasta is loaded with other tasty flavors and herbs for a perfect Mediterranean taste.

Ingredients

- Freshly cracked black pepper
- 1 lb.. short pasta
- 6 tablespoons of pine nuts, lightly toasted
- 2 cups of packed fresh basil leaves
- Kosher salt
- Zest and juice of 2 lemons
- 3 cups of grated Parmesan cheese
- 12 ounces of frozen broccoli

- 1 cup of [extra virgin olive oil](#)

Directions

- Boil water in a large pot and salt.
- Add the broccoli and cook until crisp tender in 4 minutes.
- Transfer the broccoli to a large bowl of ice water. Reserve and cooking water for later.
- Drain and dry on a paper towel.
- In the bowl of a food processor, combine the broccoli, 4 tablespoon of the pine nuts, basil leaves, Parmesan, and lemon zest and juice.
- Process until combined.
- Scrape down the sides of the bowl, run the processor again.

- Slowly stream in the extra virgin olive oil as the processor is still running.
- Season with salt and pepper.
- Bring the same pot of water back to a boil.
- Then, add the pasta, cook as per the package Directions.
- Drain the pasta and reserve some water.
- Return the drained pasta to the pot over medium heat.
- Add 1 cup of the Parmesan cheese with the reserved pasta water, let cook as you stir constantly for 1 minute.
- Remove from heat source, then add half of the broccoli pesto. Toss.
- Transfer the pasta to a large serving bowl.
- Top with the remaining Parmesan cheese and pine nuts or lemon juice.
- Serve and enjoy when garnished with basil leaves.

Stuffed tomato recipe

The stuffed tomato recipe derives its aromatic flavor from garlic and onions among other tasty spices and it makes a perfect Mediterranean Sea diet stuffed recipe.

Ingredients

- 6 large tomatoes
- 1 large red onion halved, minced
- 1 teaspoon of ground cumin
- 4 garlic cloves, minced
- ½ lb.. lean ground beef
- Kosher salt and black pepper
- ½ teaspoon of allspice
- Extra virgin olive oil
- 2 cups of canned crushed tomatoes
- ½ cup of white wine
- ½ teaspoon of ground nutmeg
- ¼ cup of water
- ½ cup long grain rice
- ¾ teaspoon of dried oregano
- 1 cup of chopped fresh parsley
- ½ cup of chopped fresh spearmint

Directions

- Place the rice in a bowl and cover with water.
- Soak for 20 minutes until it is easy to break one grain of rice between your fingertips.
- Drain any excess water.
- Preheat your oven to 375°F.

- Place a large skillet over medium-high heat.
- Add ⅓ cup of extra virgin olive oil let heat until just shimmering but with no smoke.
- Add chopped onions together with the garlic, toss until fragrant.
- Add the ground meat, season with salt, pepper, cumin, oregano, nutmeg, and allspice and let cook for 5 minutes or until fully browned.
- Add drained rice it to the meat mixture in the skillet.
- Add crushed tomatoes together with the white wine and water.
- Bring the saucy mixture to a boil, lower the heat let simmer for 10 minutes.
- Stir in the fresh herbs.
- Season with kosher salt.
- Cut tomato tops and keep the tops aside.
- Loosen the tomatoes with a knife by going around the edges of the tomato.
- Scoop out the tomato flesh and chop the flesh into large pieces, keep for later.
- Prepare a baking pan by oiling the bottom with extra virgin olive oil.
- Spread the chopped tomato flesh and sliced onion at the bottom of the baking dish.
- Add the chopped tomato flesh together with the sliced onion to make a bed for the stuffed tomatoes.

- Spoon the saucy meat and rice mixture into the empty tomato shells.
- Organize the stuffed tomatoes in the prepared baking dish.
- Cover with the reserved tops.
- From one of the corners of your baking dish, carefully pour ¾ cup of water.
- Add a little pinch of salt and a generous drizzle of extra virgin olive oil on top.
- Cover the baking dish with foil let bake in heated oven for 45 minutes.
- Let cook uncovered for more 45 minutes.
- Let cool.
- Serve and enjoy.

Classic tiramisu

This mighty classic tiramisu features ladyfingers dipped in espresso together with Kahlua layer of a mascarpone custard fluffy with tasty cream.

Ingredients

- 8 ounces of mascarpone cheese at room temperature
- ½ cup plus 2 tablespoons of Kahlua liqueur
- 1 teaspoon of vanilla extract
- 3 eggs
- ½ cup of granulated sugar divided
- 1 cup of boiling water
- 1 7- ounce package of Savoiardi cookies
- Cocoa powder
- 4 cups of whipping cream
- 6 tablespoons of instant espresso powder

Directions

- Bring 1 cup of water to a boil.
- Pour into a shallow bowl.
- Mix in the espresso powder and ½ cup of the Kahlua liqueur. Set aside to cool.
- Separate the egg yolks from the whites, make sure to save the whites.
- Add the yolks to a small, heat proof bowl that fits snugly over another saucepan filled with about 2 inches of water.

- Let the water simmer gently and top with the bowl of egg yolks.
- Add ¼ cup of sugar to the egg yolks, use a hand mixer to beat the eggs on medium speed over the simmering water for 5 minutes until the mixtures is creamy and light yellow.
- Remove the bowl from the heat, let cool.
- In another large bowl, add the whipping cream, remaining ¼ cup of sugar, 2 tablespoons Kahlua and the vanilla, beat until stiff peaks form.
- Shift the cooled egg yolk mixture to a large bowl.
- Add the mascarpone to the egg yolk mixture and blend until smooth.
- Gently fold the whipping cream into the egg yolk mixture with a large spatula.
- Toss the ladyfingers in the espresso mixture and arrange half of them in a single layer in the bottom of a pan.
- Spread half of the whipped cream mixture over the ladyfingers.
- Let soak the remaining ladyfingers 3 at a time to create another layer and top with the remaining whip cream mixture and spread equally over the top.
- Cover with plastic wrap and refrigerate for at 8 hours up to 48 hours.
- Run a knife along the inside of the pan and cut into squares.

- Dust the servings with cocoa powder and serve.
- Enjoy.

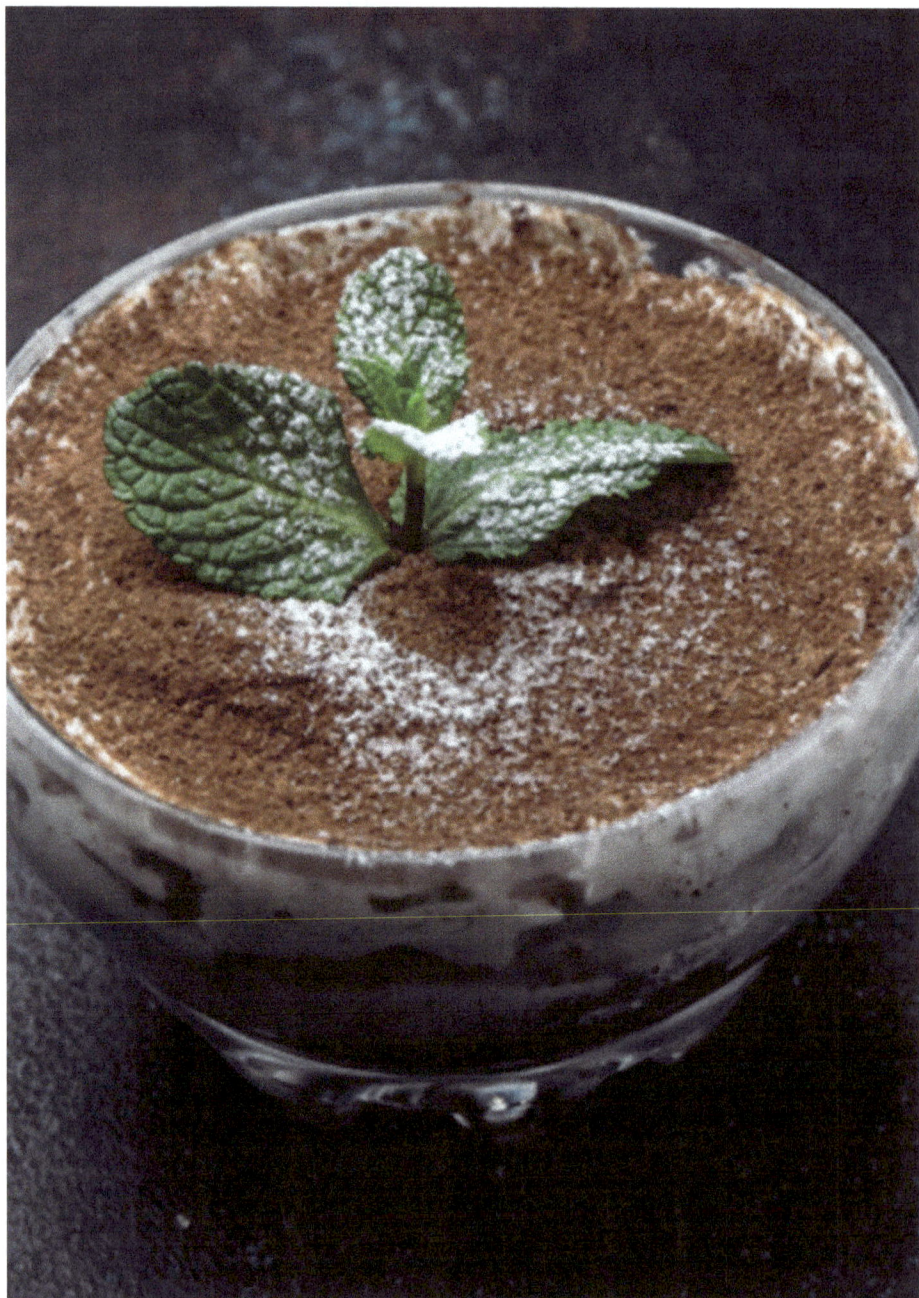

Za'atar manaquish recipe

The eastern Mediterranean region makes this recipe as their favorite featuring vegetables and tasty and aromatic spices.

Ingredients

- 1 cup of lukewarm water
- Radish
- ½ cup of extra virgin olive oil
- ½ teaspoon of sugar
- 3 cups unbleached all-purpose flour,
- Feta cheese
- Cucumbers
- 1 tsp salt
- 2 tablespoons of extra virgin olive oil
- 8 tablespoons of quality [Za'atar spice](#)
- 2 ¼ teaspoons of active dry yeast
- Tomatoes
- Olives

Directions

- Preheat your oven to 400°F. Place a large baking sheet in oven while heating
- In a small bowl, combine water, sugar and yeast. Keep for 10 minutes to let foam.
- In another separate large mixing bowl, combine flour together with salt, and olive oil.
- Work the mixture with your hands.

- Make a well in the middle and pour in the yeast and water mixture. Stir until soft dough forms.
- Turn dough onto a lightly floured surface and knead for 10 minutes or until dough is elastic, smooth.
- Form dough into a ball and place in a lightly oiled mixing bowl.
- Cover with damp cloth and place in a warm spot and let rise for 2 hours.
- Punch dough down. Knead briefly and form into 8 small balls.
- Organize on lightly floured surface, cover again and leave to rise for more 30 minutes.
- Next, mix together the za'atar spice and olive oil in a bowl.
- Lightly oil the heated baking sheet and set close.
- Flatten the dough into small discs.
- Make indentations in discs.
- Add 1 tablespoon of za'atar topping in the middle of each disc, leave a narrow boarder around.
- Organize the discs in prepared oiled baking sheet.
- Bake in the preheated-oven for 8 minutes.
- Remove from heat and let sit for 5 minutes.
- Topping will dry and settle into dough.
- Serve za'atar manaquish warm with assorted vegetables.
- Enjoy.

Mediterranean style bean dip with roasted squash

Ingredients

- Extra virgin olive oil
- ¾ teaspoon of ground coriander
- 2 tablespoons of toasted pine nuts for garnish
- 2 shallots, peeled and thinly sliced
- ¾ teaspoon of ground cumin
- 2 tablespoons of toasted slivered almonds
- 2 teaspoon of fresh lemon juice
- 1 15-oz. can of cannellini beans, drained and rinsed
- 1 garlic clove, chopped
- ¾ teaspoon of Spanish paprika
- 1 Acorn squash
- ½ teaspoon of cayenne pepper
- Flat leaf parsley for garnish
- ¾ teaspoon of ground sumac

Directions

- Start by preheating your oven to 400°F.
- Place acorn squash in microwave and heat on high for 3 minutes.
- Cut the acorn squash in half through the stem.
- Scoop out the seeds using a spoon.
- Sprinkle the squash with salt, put them flesh side down on a lightly oiled baking sheet.

- Roast in the preheated oven for 40 minutes until flesh is tender and slightly browned.
- In a skillet, heat 1 tablespoon of extra virgin olive oil over medium-high.
- Add the shallots and let sauté until caramelized, keep tossing regularly.
- Season with salt.
- Remove squash from the oven let cool down.
- Scoop out the flesh and discard shell.
- In the bowl of a large food processor, add ½ amount of shallots, squash, white beans, all the spices and then sprinkle with a pinch of salt.
- Add lemon juice and 3 tablespoon of extra virgin olive oil.
- Then, close the top of your processor let blend until desired a smooth dip.
- Taste and adjust accordingly.
- Shift the dip to a serving bowl.
- Add a drizzle of olive oil together with the parsley leaves and toasted nuts.
- Serve and enjoy with warm pita.

Egyptian koshari recipe

Egyptian koshari recipe as the name suggests, it is a typical Egyptian Mediterranean recipe with variety of vegetables especially, onions, tomatoes, garlic for tasty aromatic flavor.

Ingredients

- ½ teaspoon of crushed red pepper flakes
- 1 can of 28-oz. tomato sauce
- ⅓ cup of all-purpose flour
- ½ cup of cooking oil
- 1 teaspoon of ground coriander
- Cooking oil
- 1 small onion, grated
- 1 large onion, sliced into thin rings
- 2 tablespoons of distilled white vinegar
- 4 garlic cloves, minced
- Salt and pepper
- Salt

For Koshari

- 1 15-oz. can of chickpeas, rinsed, drained and warmed
- Water
- ½ teaspoon of each salt and pepper
- ½ teaspoon of coriander
- 1 ½ cup brown lentils, picked over and well-rinsed
- Cooking oil
- 1 ½ cup medium-grain rice, rinsed, soaked

- 2 cups of elbow pasta

Directions

- Sprinkle the onion rings with salt, then toss them in the flour to coat. Shake off any excess flour.
- In a large skillet, heat cooking oil over medium heat, cook the onion rings, stirring often, until caramelized brown within 18 minutes.
- In a saucepan, heat 1 tablespoon of cooking oil.
- Add the grated onion, cook on medium until the onion turns a translucent.
- Add the garlic together with the coriander, and red pepper flakes, then sauté until fragrant in 45 seconds.
- Stir in tomato sauce and pinch of salt.
- Let simmer over low heat until the sauce thickens in 15 minutes.
- Stir in the distilled white vinegar, and turn the heat to low.
- Cover and keep warm.
- Bring lentils to boil with 4 cups of water in a medium pot over high heat.
- Lower the heat let continue to cook until lentils are just tender.
- Drain any excess water.
- Season with a little salt.
- Drain the rice from its soaking water.

- Combine the par-cooked lentils and the rice in the saucepan over medium heat with 1 tablespoon of cooking oil, salt, pepper, and coriander.
- For 3 minutes, let cook while stirring regularly.
- Add warm water to cover the rice and lentil mixture.
- Bring to a boil let the water reduce a little.
- Cover continue to cook to absorb excess liquid and both the rice and lentils are well cooked in 20 minutes.
- Let it rest undisturbed and covered for 5 minutes.
- Make the pasta accordingly to the manufacturers package Directions.
- Drain any excess water.
- Cover the chickpeas and warm in the microwave shortly.
- Next, fluff the rice and lentils with a fork.
- Shift to a serving platter.
- Then, Top with the elbow pasta and tomato sauce, chickpeas also crispy onions for purposes of garnishing.
- Serve and enjoy.

Mediterranean pan seared sea bass recipe with a garlic bell pepper medley

Ingredients

- ½ tablespoon of garlic powder
- 4 pieces of Sea Bass fillet, no skin
- 1 teaspoon of Aleppo pepper
- 3 cups of cooked rice
- Salt

- Extra virgin olive oil
- 1 Green Bell Pepper, cored and chopped
- 1 Red Bell Pepper, cored and chopped
- ½ lemon, juice off
- 1 teaspoon of ground cumin
- 3 Shallots, chopped
- ½ teaspoon of black pepper
- 4 garlic cloves, minced
- ½ cup of pitted Kalamata olives, halved
- ½ tablespoon of ground coriander

Directions

- Take the fish out of the fridge about 20 minutes before cooking. Sprinkle with salt on both sides and set aside.
- In a small bowl, combine the spices to make the spice mixture. Also set aside for later.
- In a medium-sized skillet, heat 2 tablespoon of olive oil over medium-high heat until shimmering but with no smoke.

- Add the bell peppers together with the shallots and garlic.
- Season with salt and spice mixture you prepared earlier.
- Let cook for 5 minutes as you stir regularly until the peppers have softened.
- Lower the heat stir in the chopped olives.
- Leave on low heat as fish gets ready.
- Pat fish dry and season with the remaining spice mixture.
- In a large skillet, heat ¼ cup of extra virgin olive oil over medium-high until shimmering but with no smoke.
- Add the fish pieces.
- Push to the middle for 30 seconds.
- Let cook on one side, undisturbed, until nicely browned not longer than 6 minutes.
- Turn the fish over and cook on other side for the same until nicely browned as well.
- Remove fish from source of heat.
- Drizzle with lemon juice.
- Serve hot and enjoy with the bell pepper medley spooned on top as well as cooked couscous.

www.ingramcontent.com/pod-product-compliance
Lightning Source LLC
Chambersburg PA
CBHW050752030426
42336CB00012B/1771